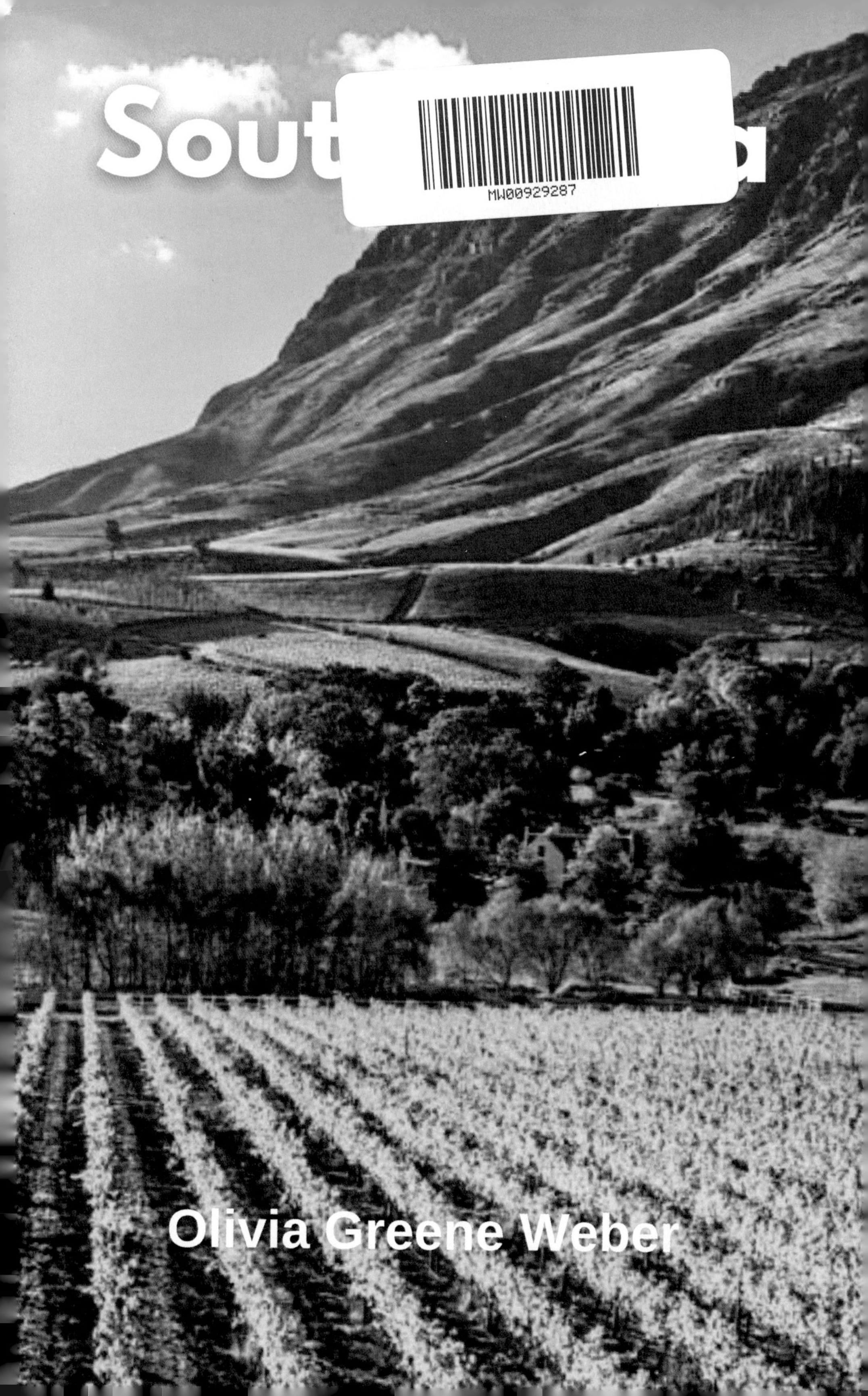

Sout[illegible]a

Olivia Greene Weber

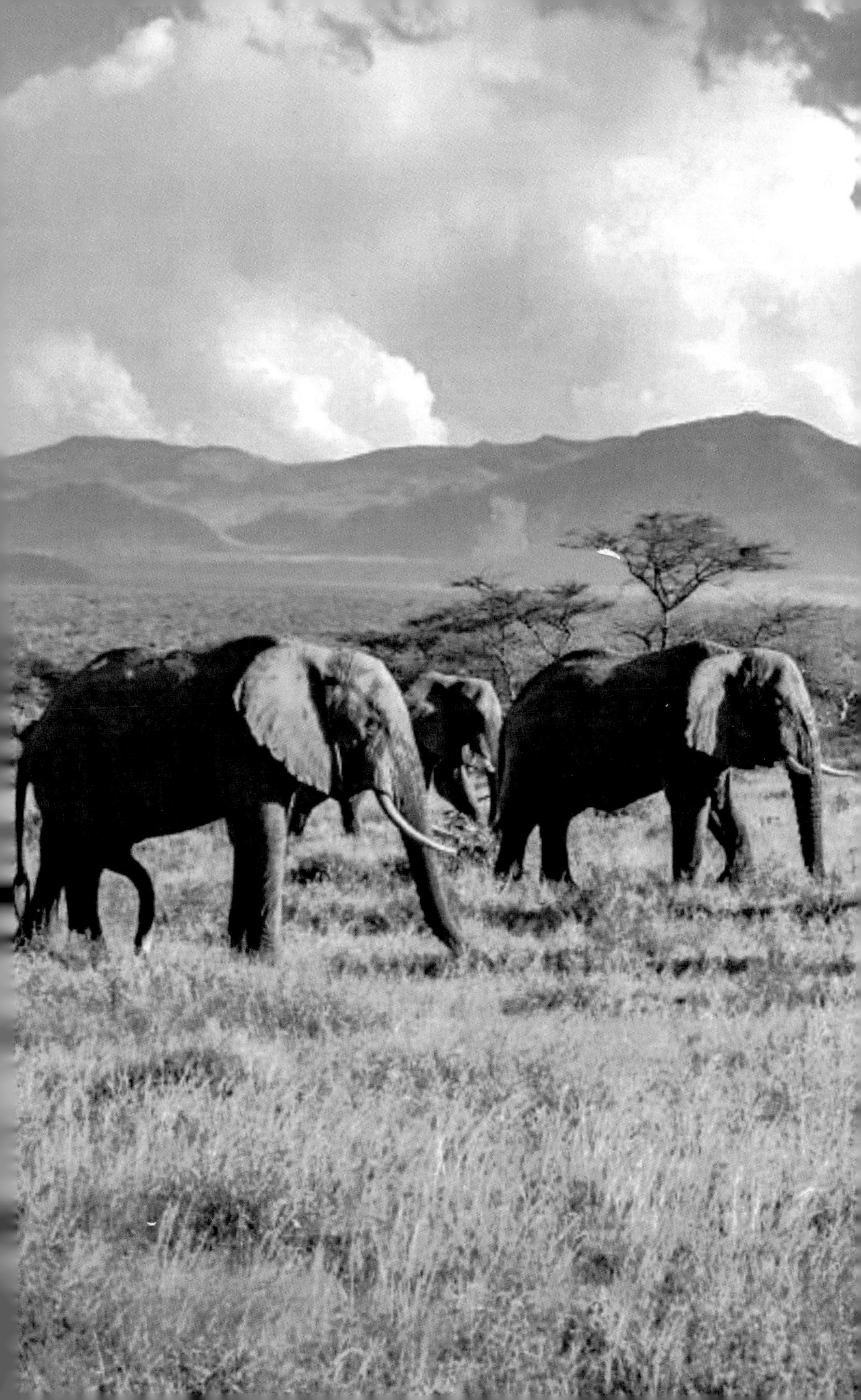

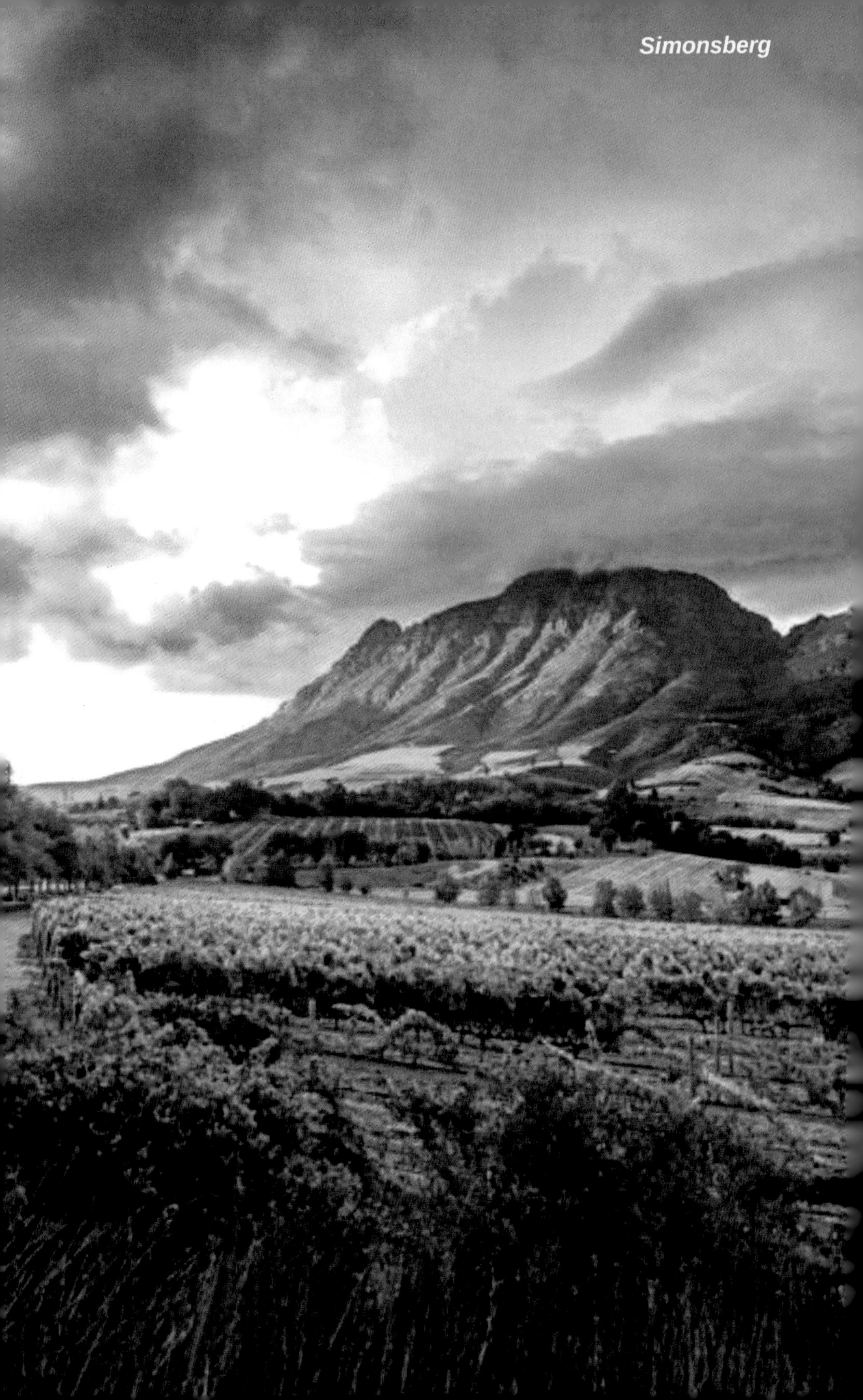

Simonsberg

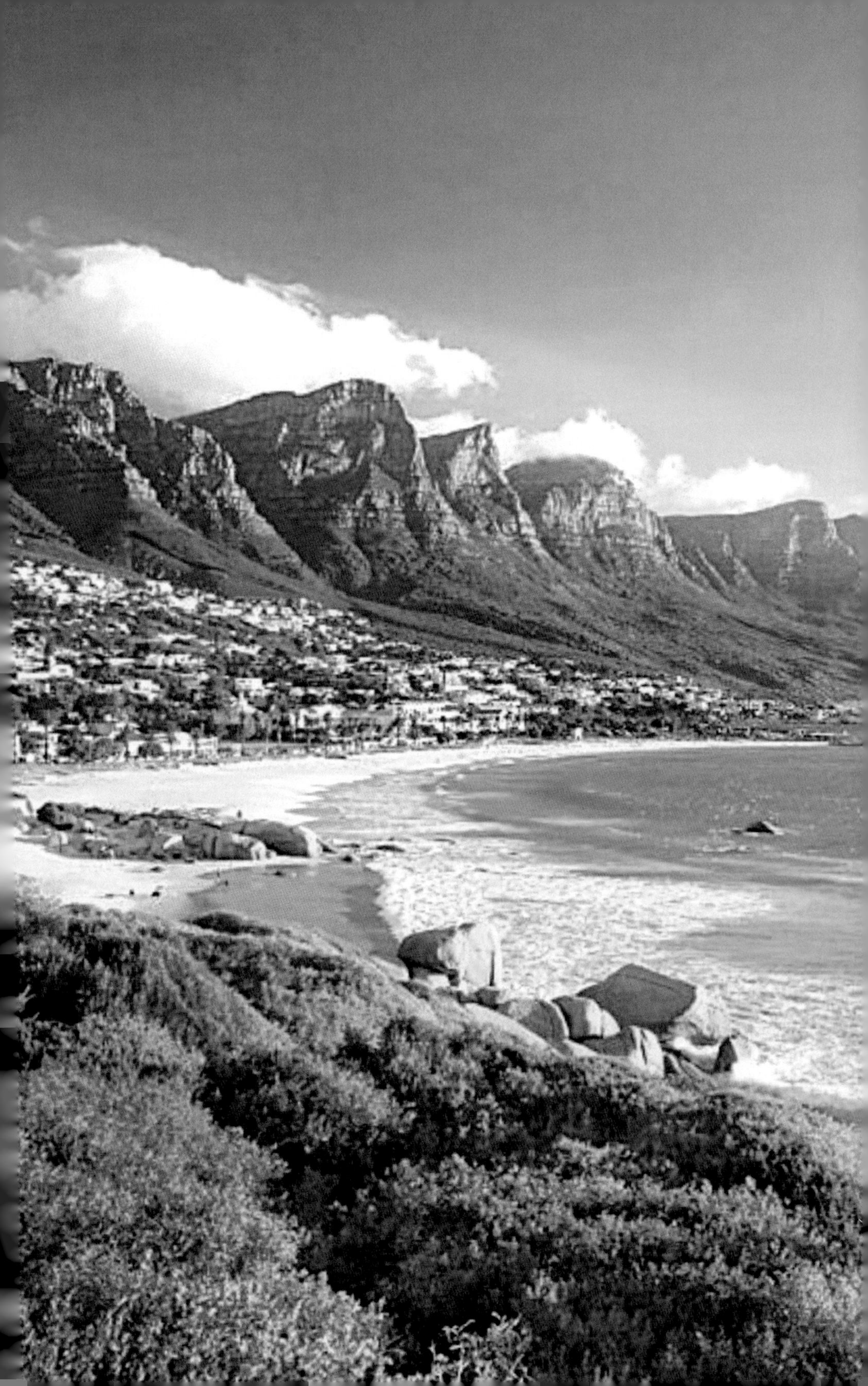

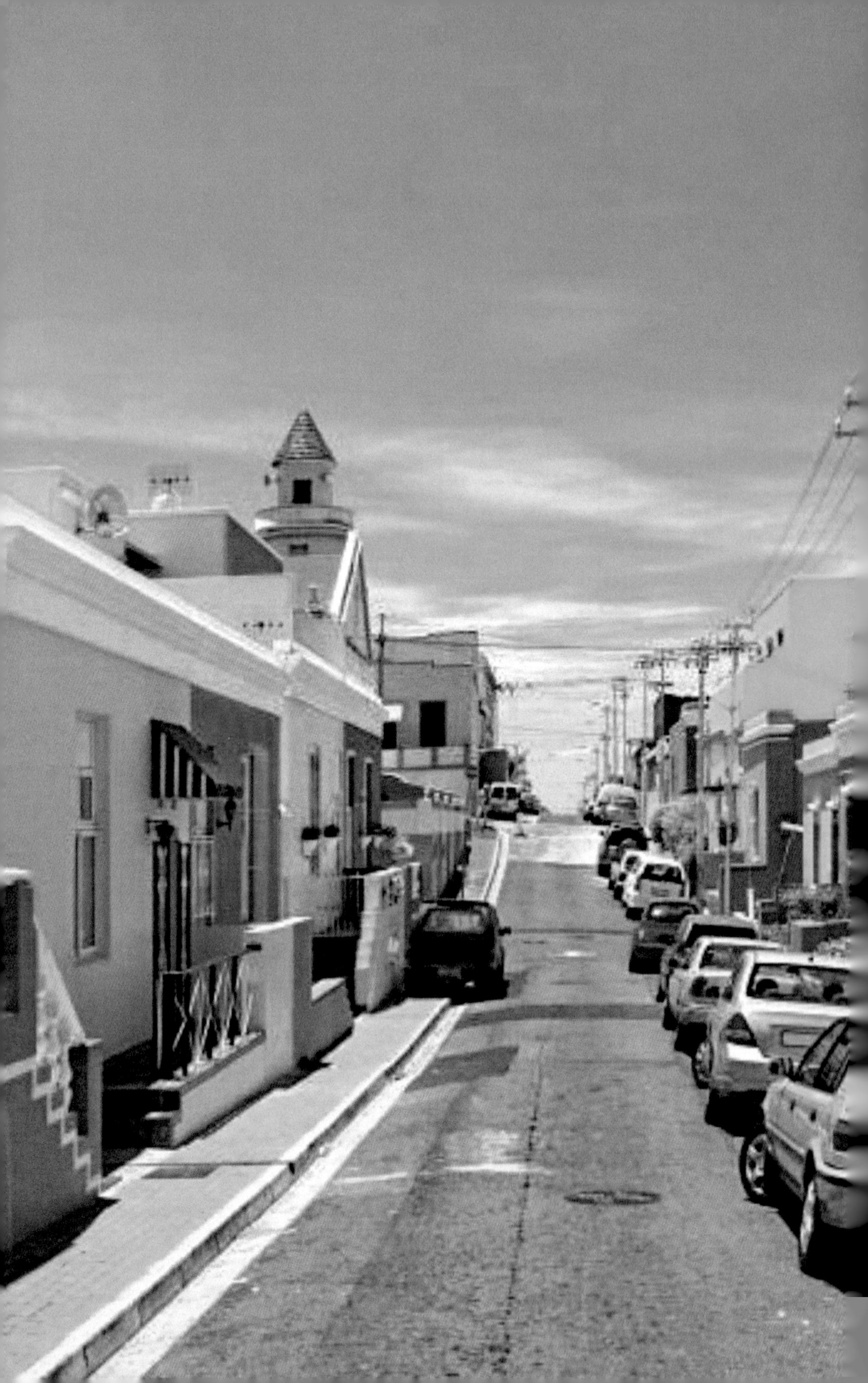

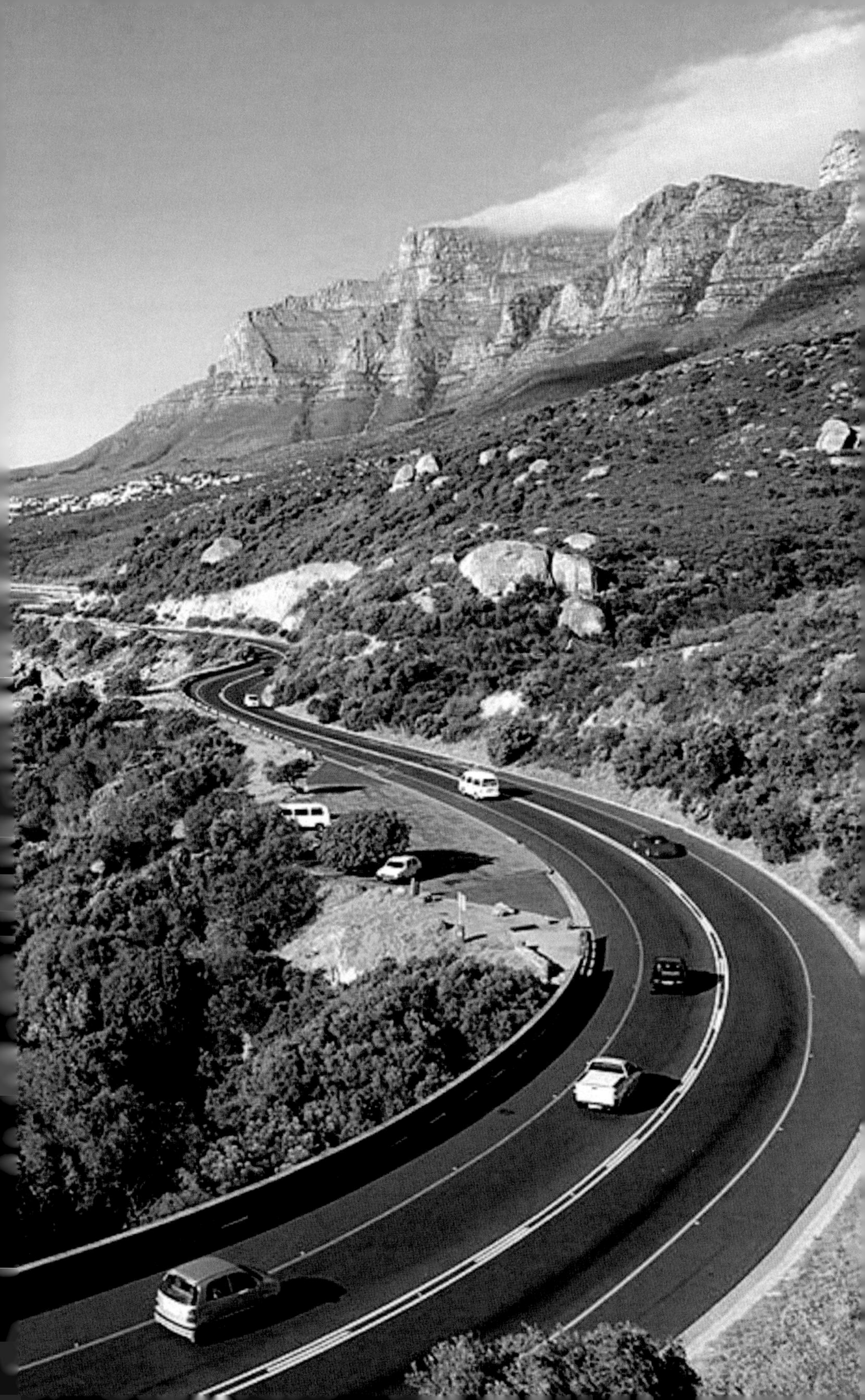

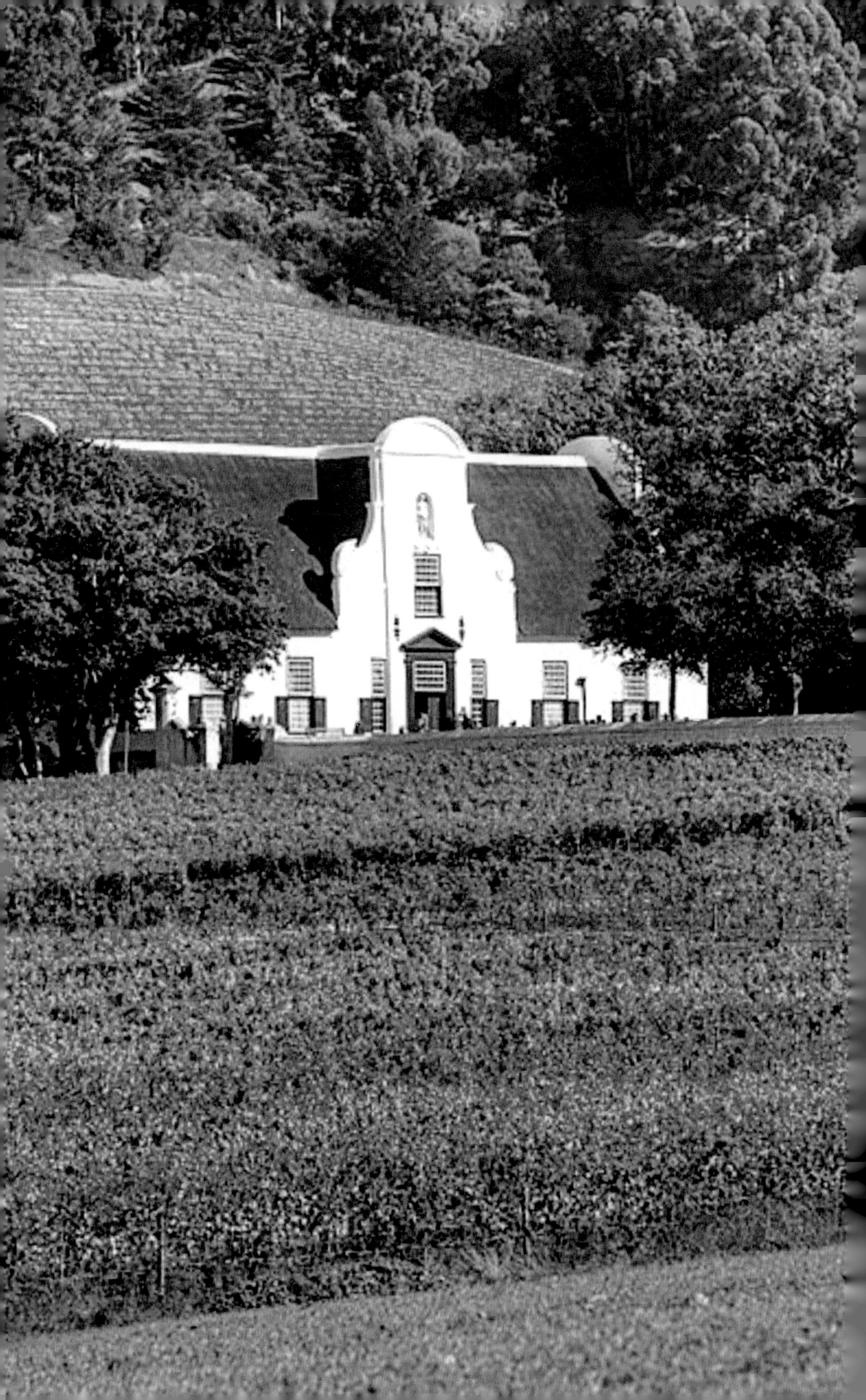

Big Hole

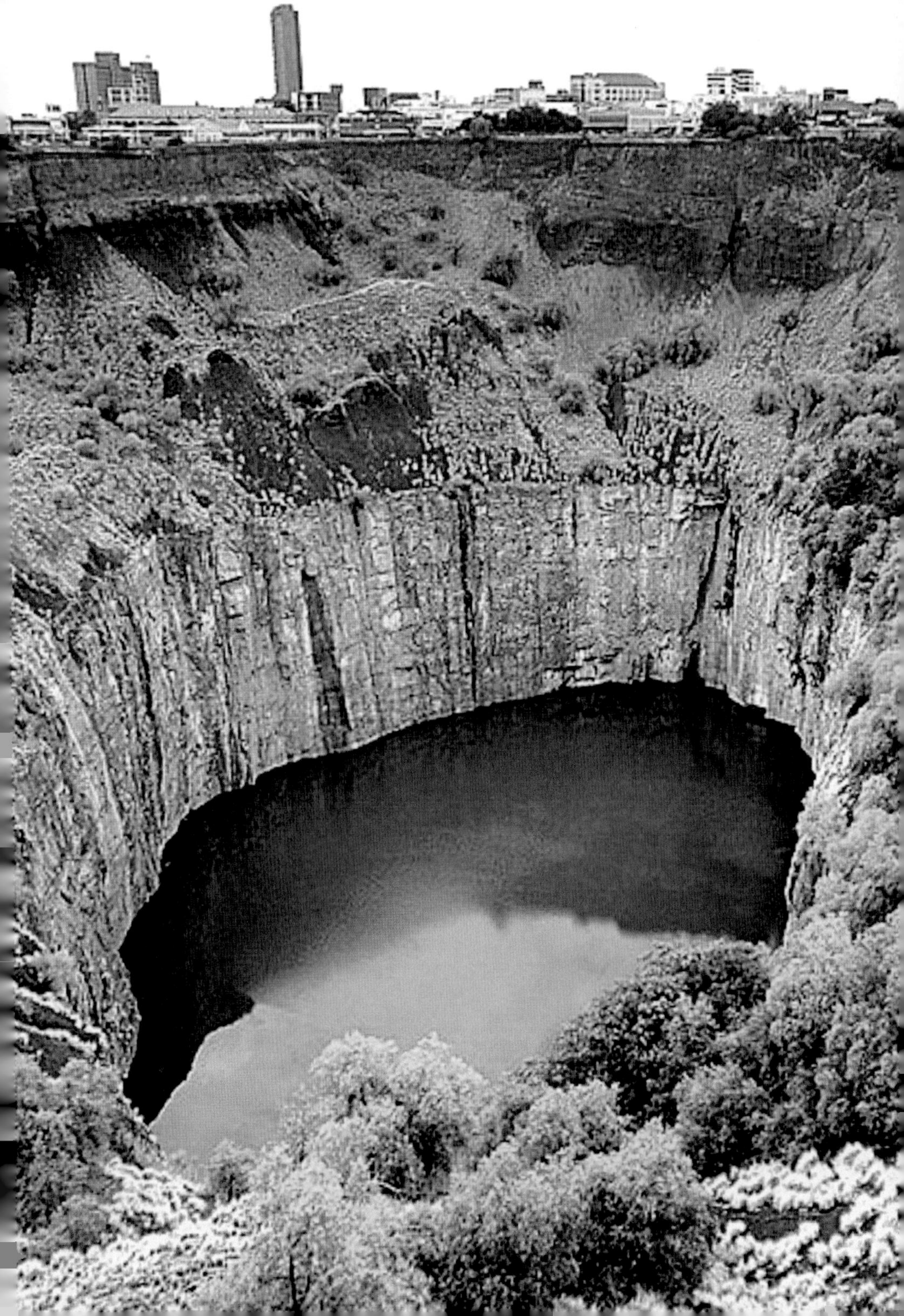

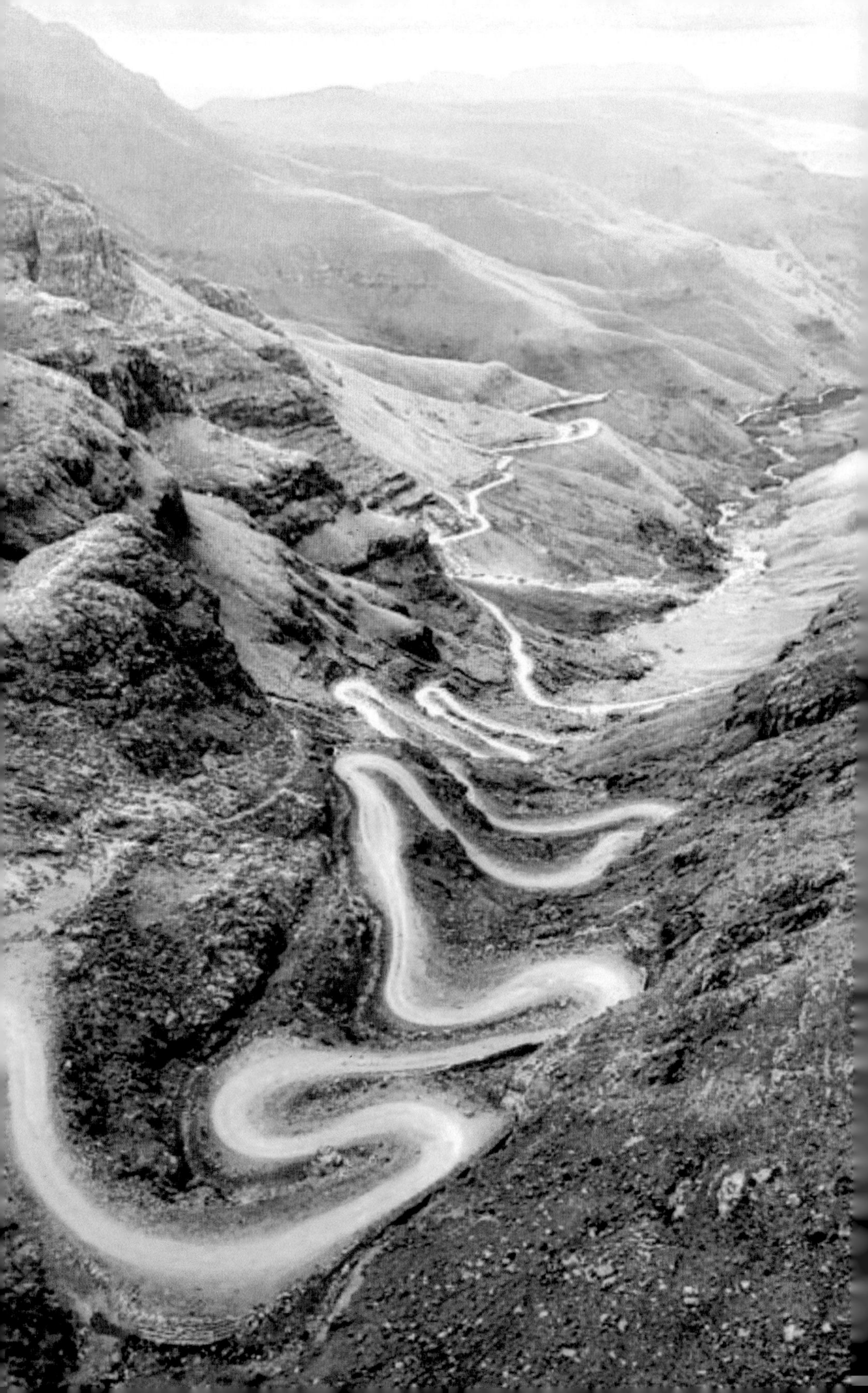

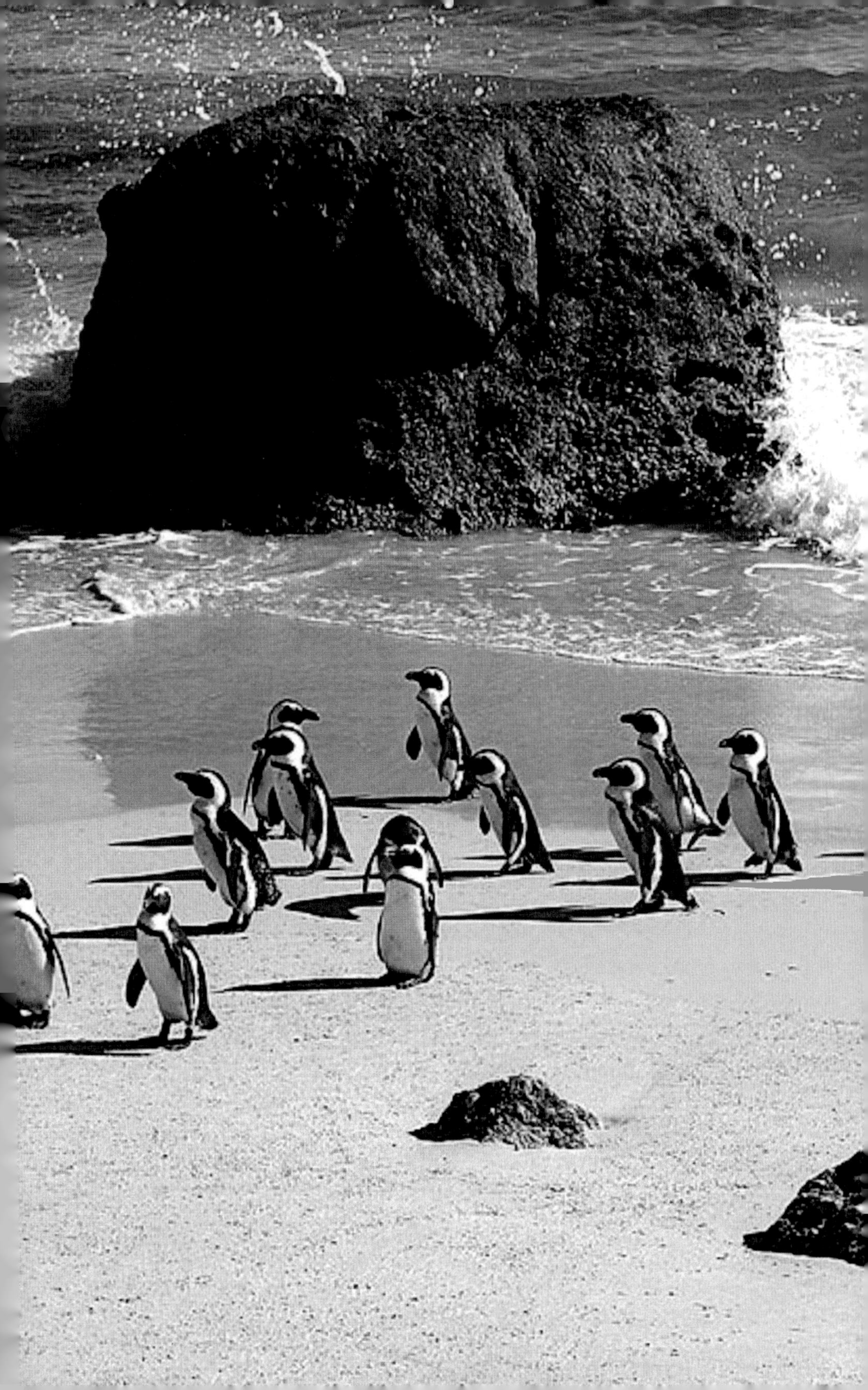

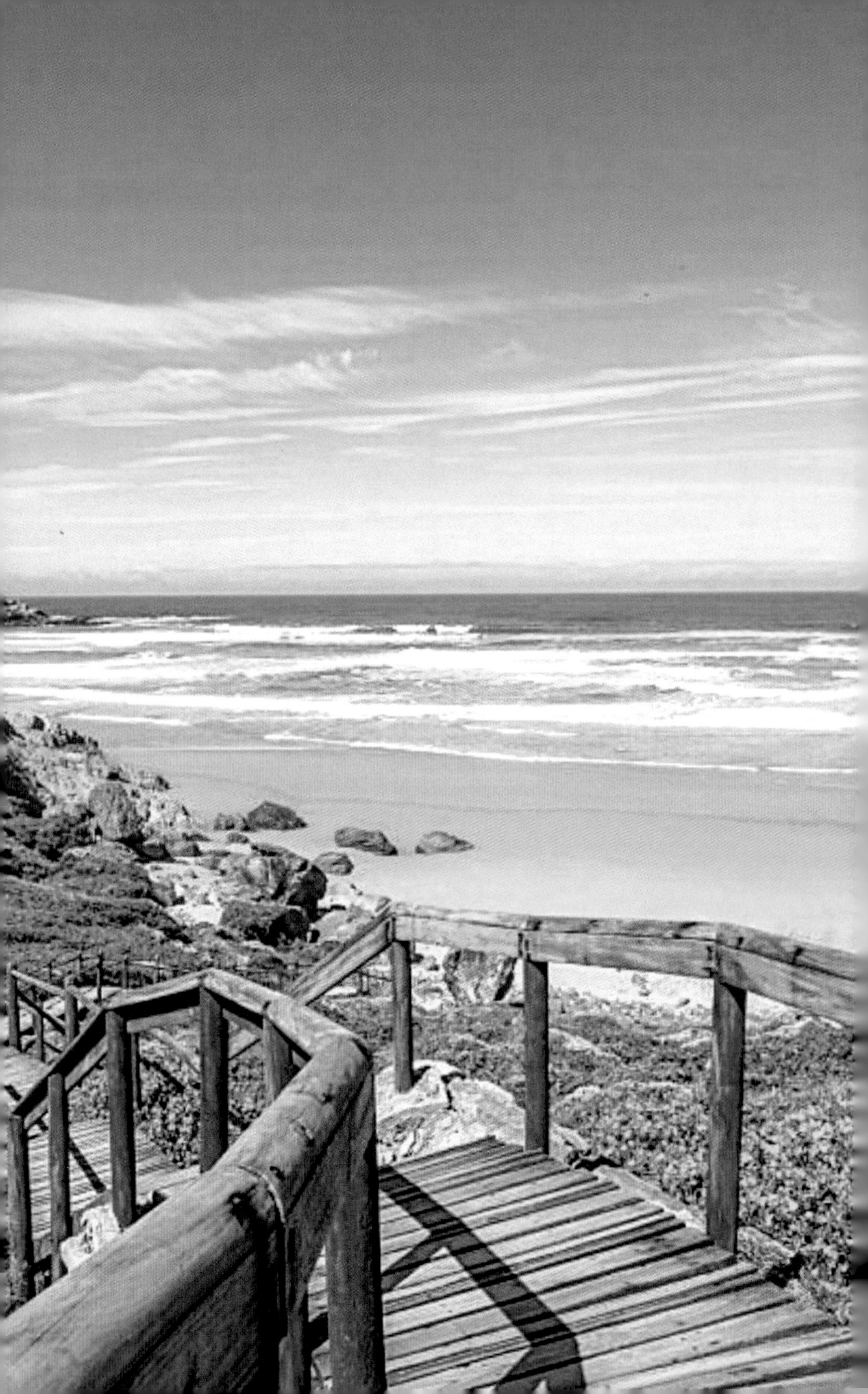

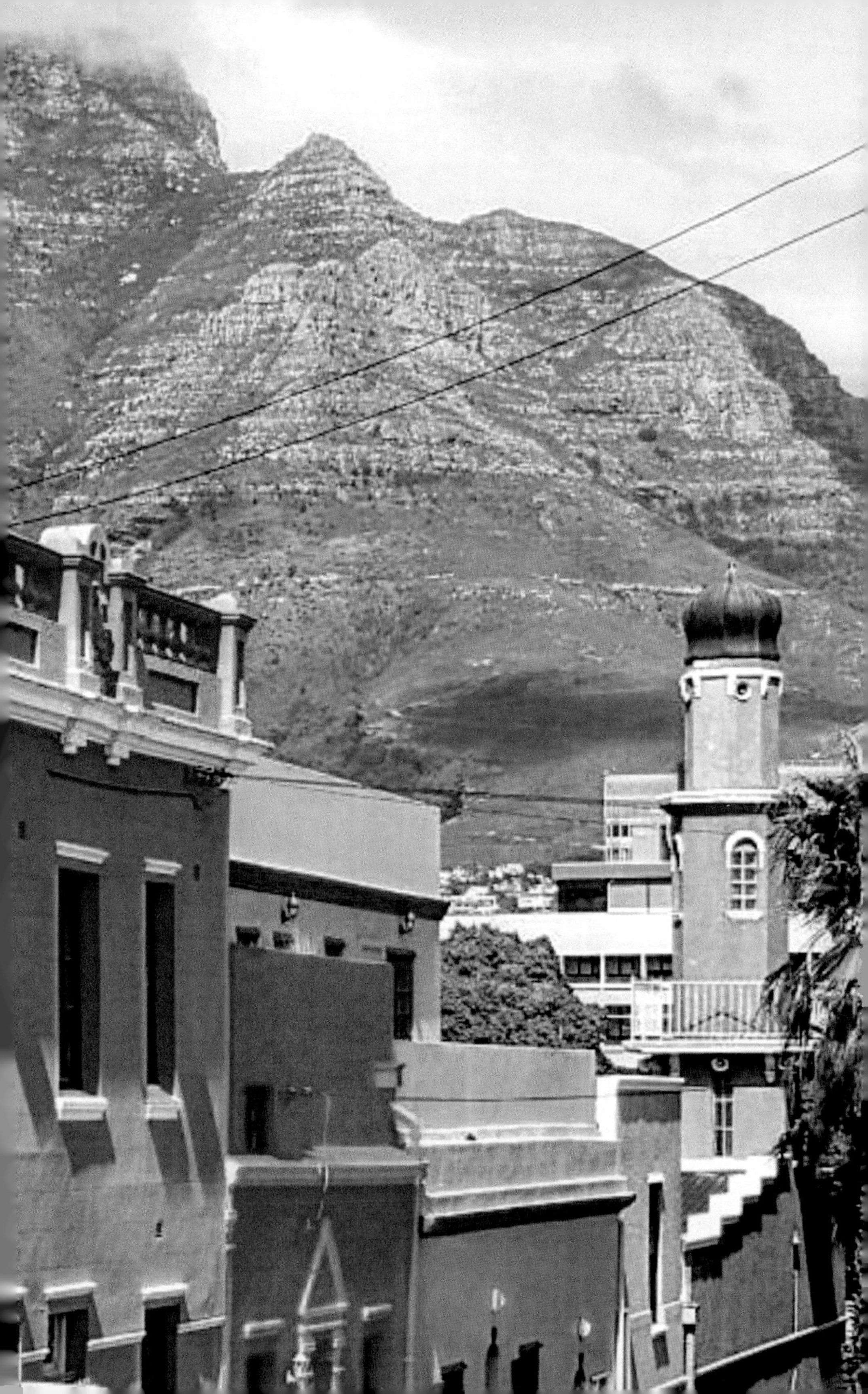

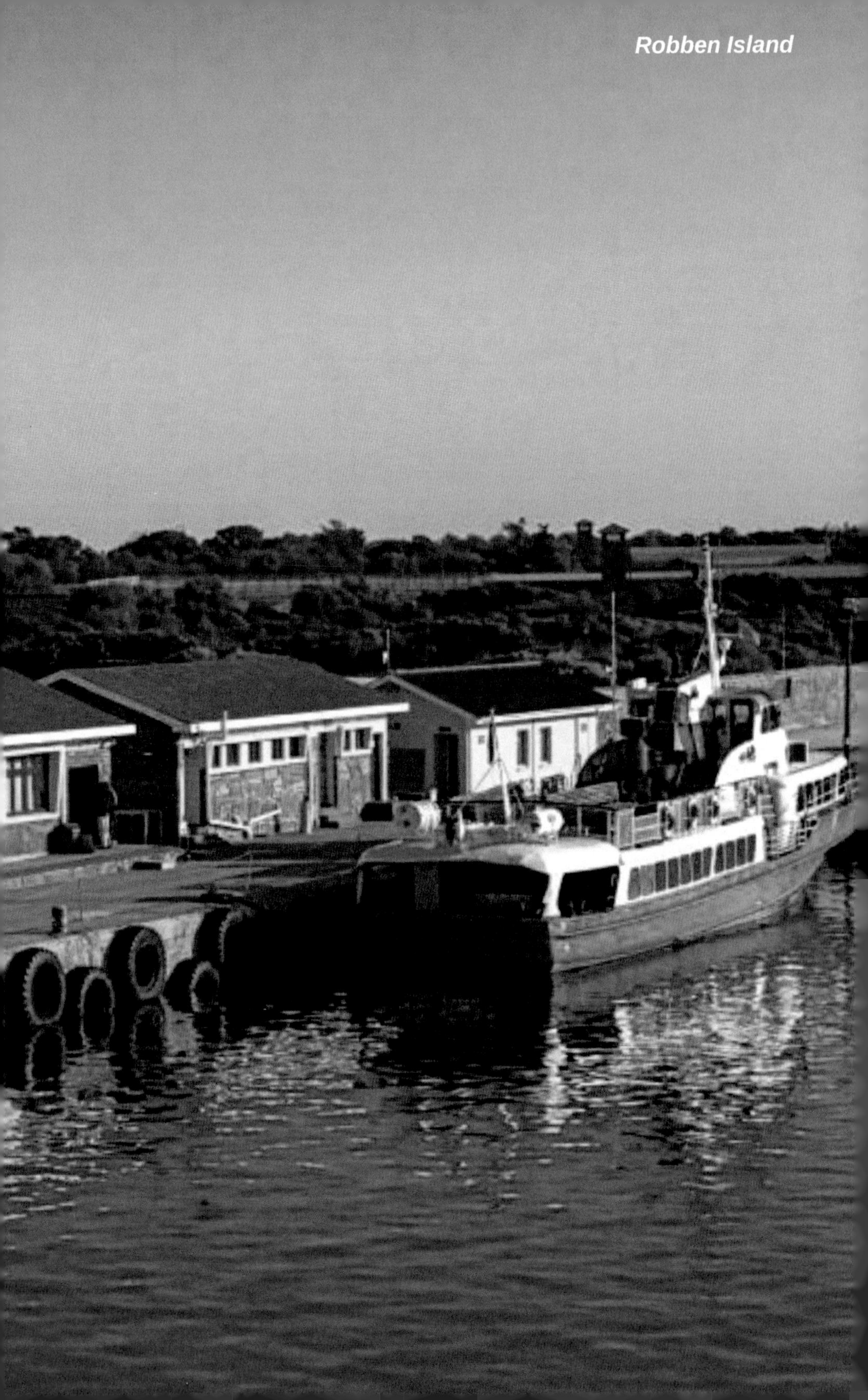
Robben Island

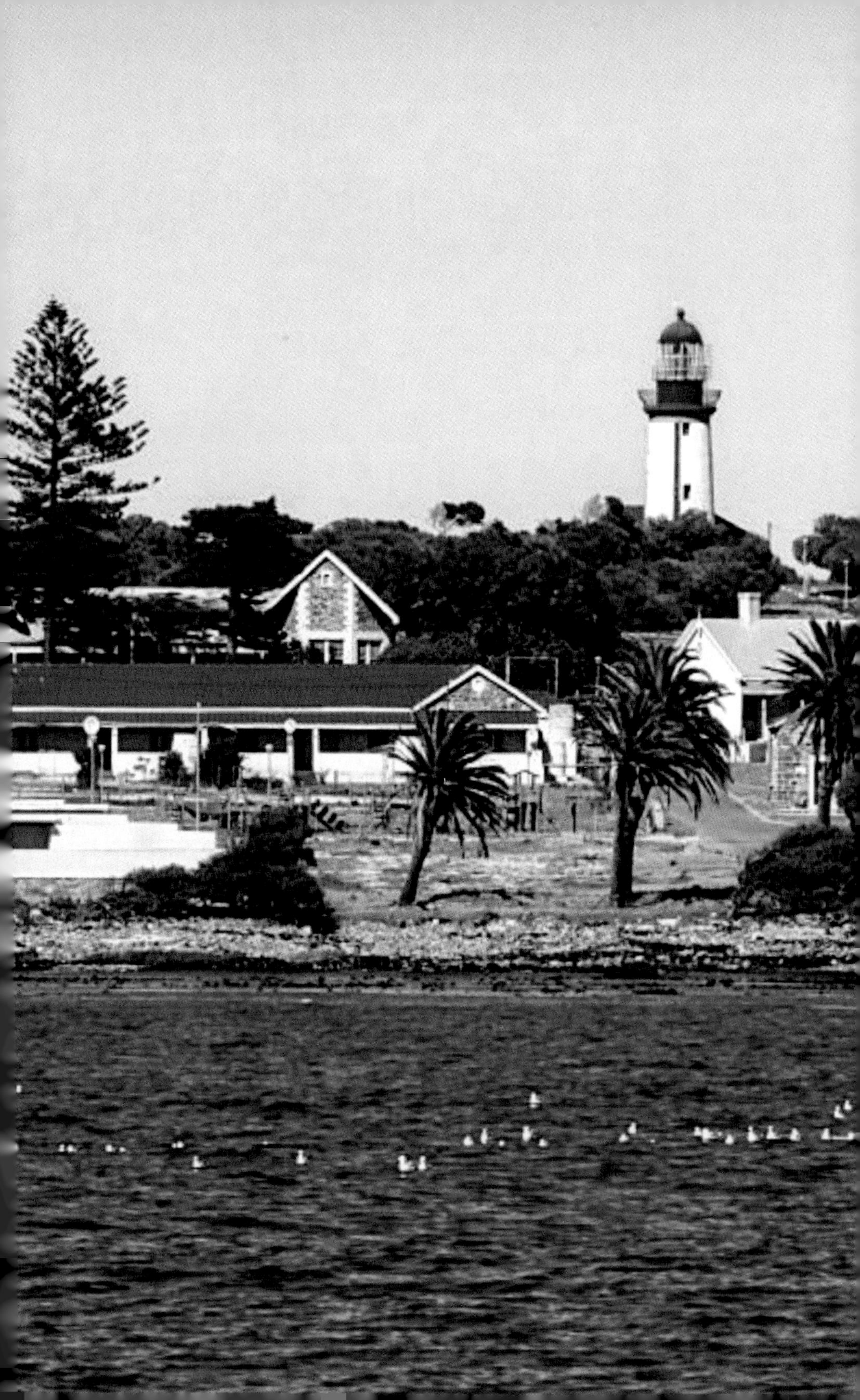

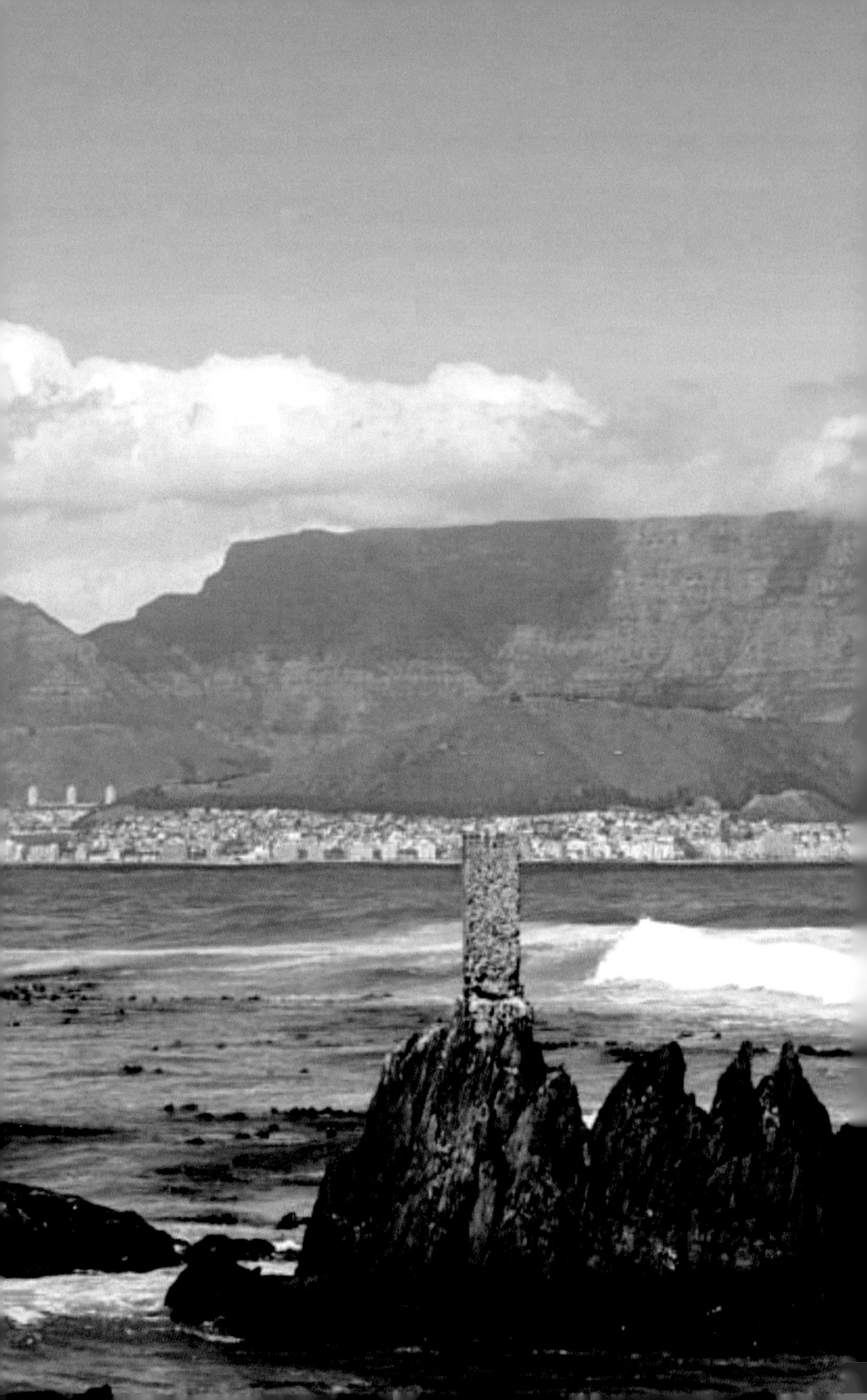

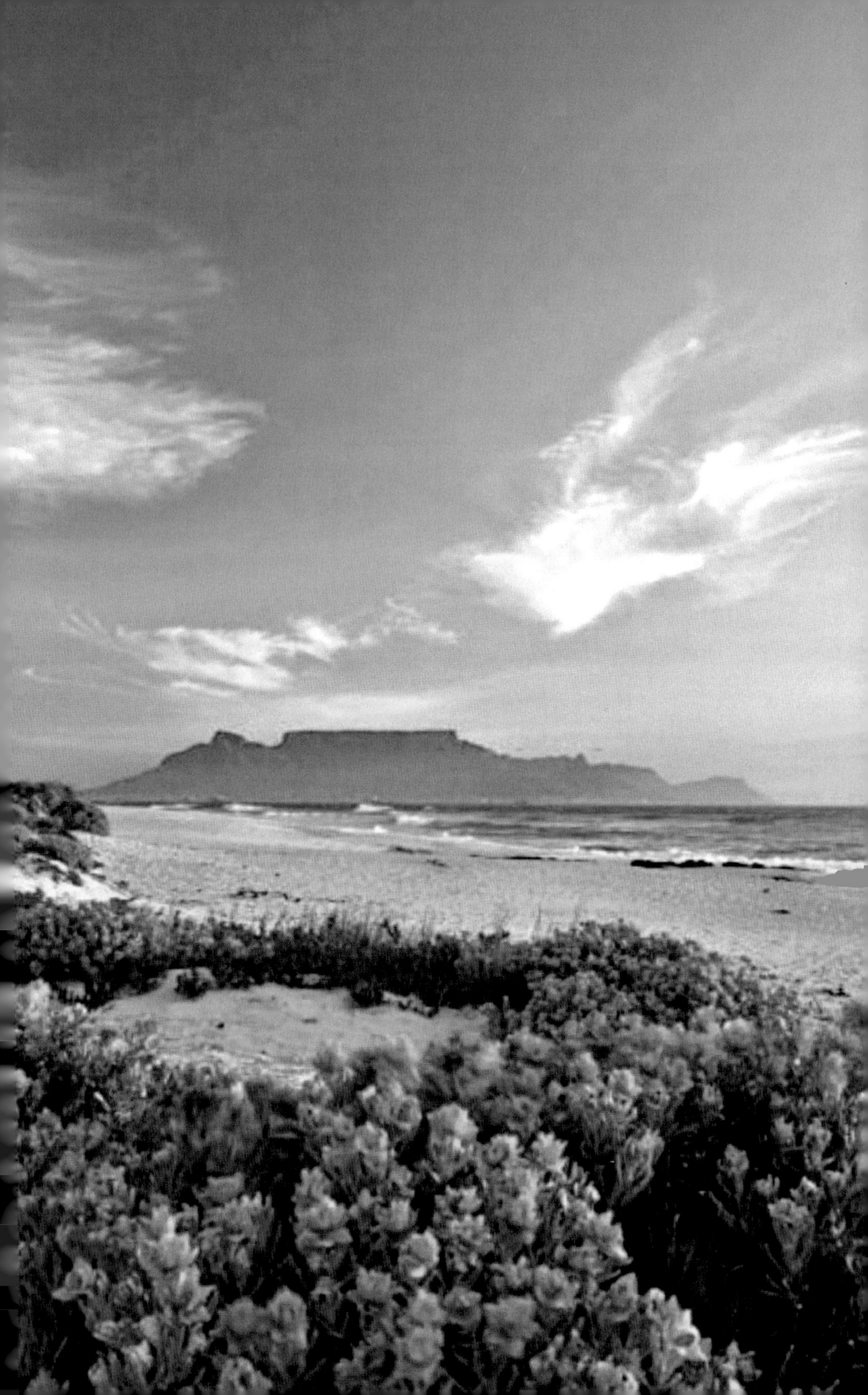

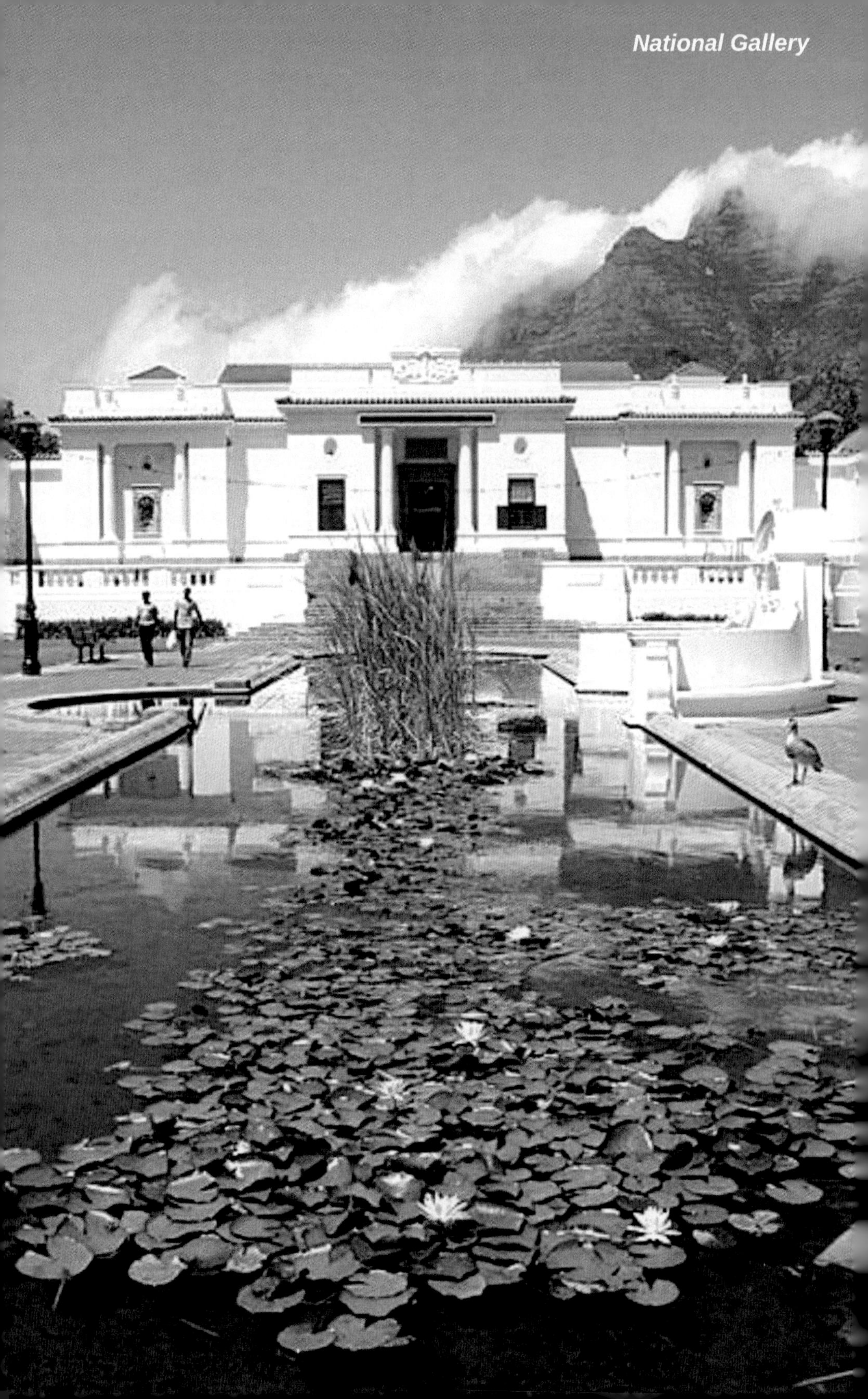
National Gallery

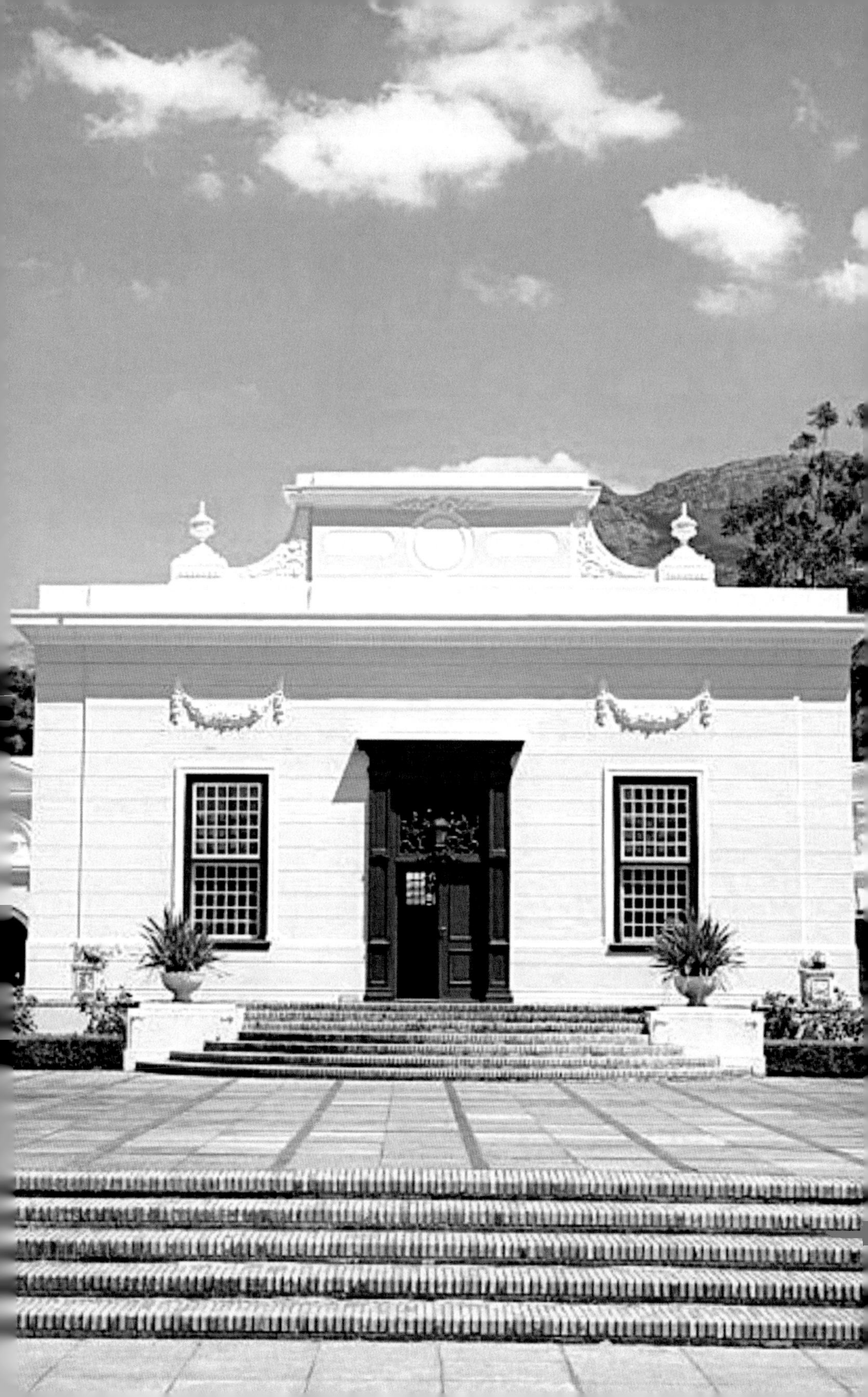

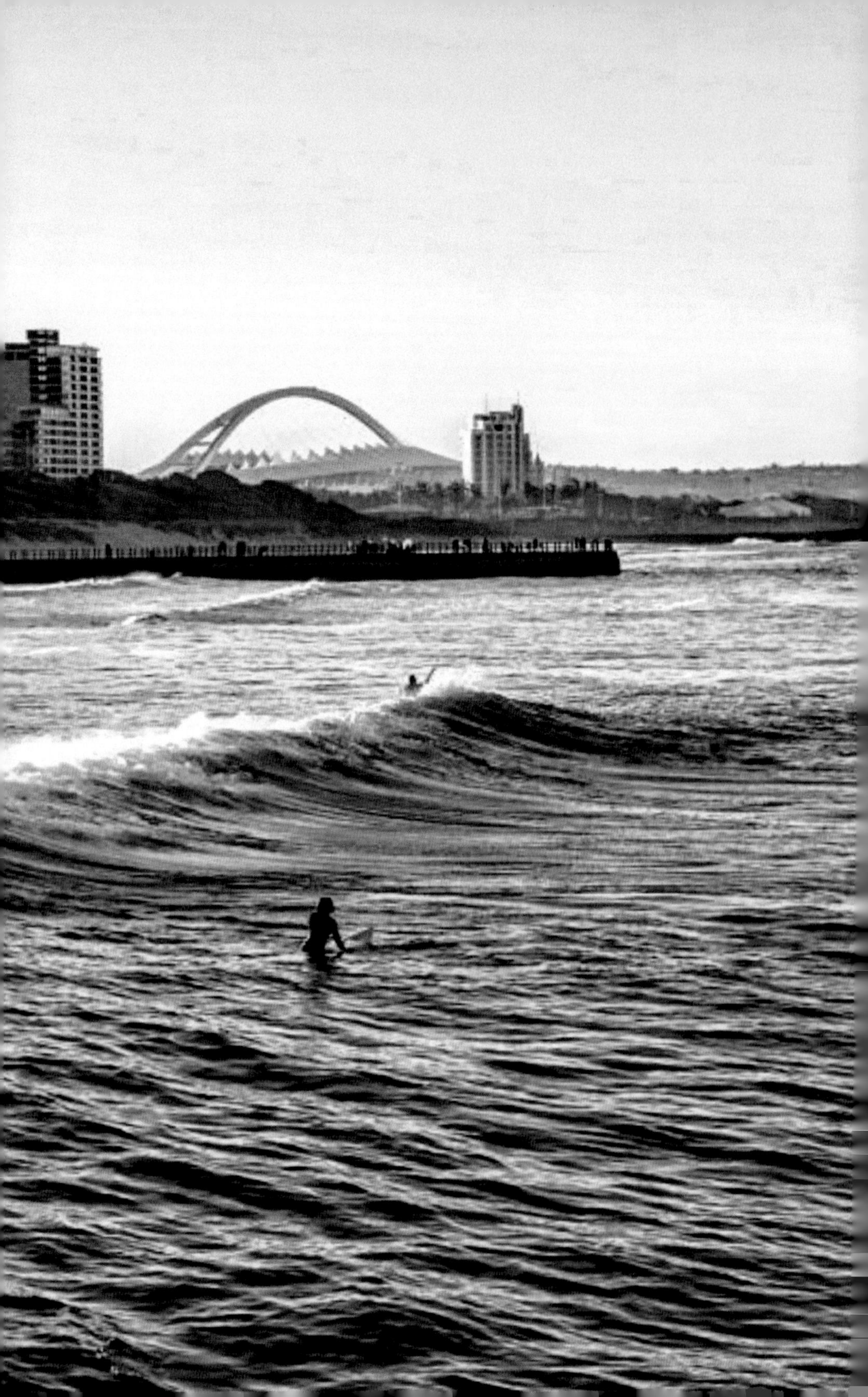

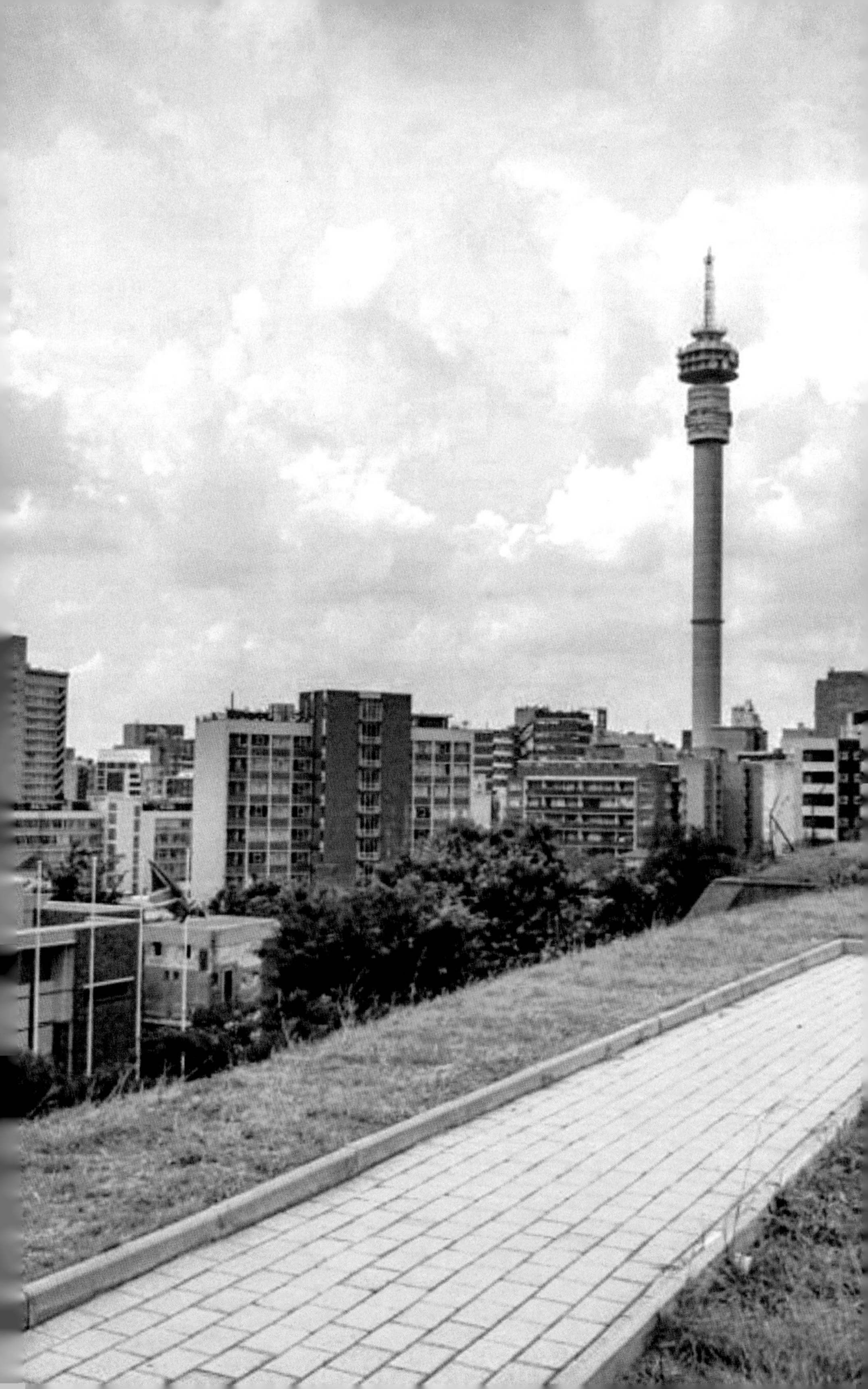

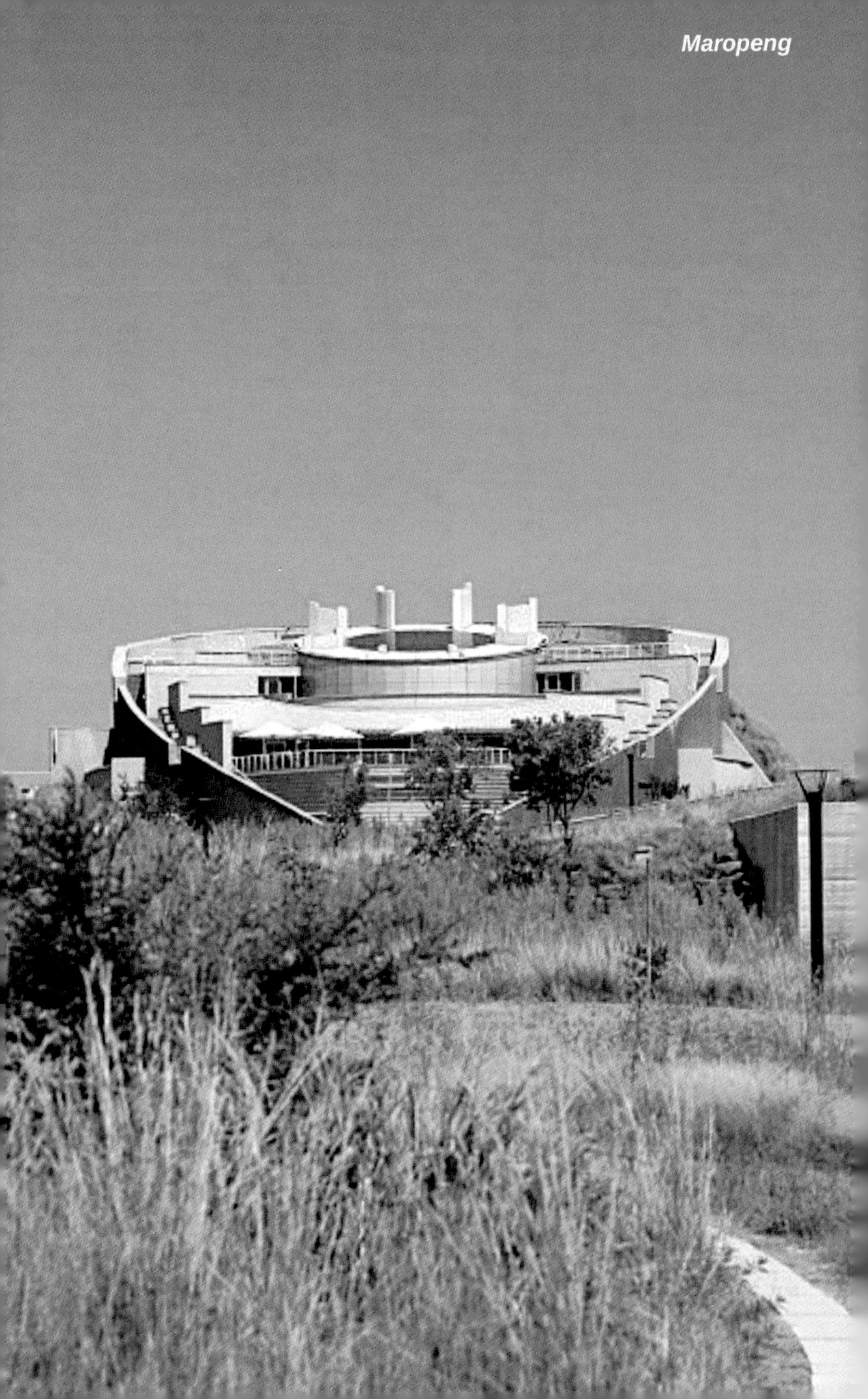

Maropeng

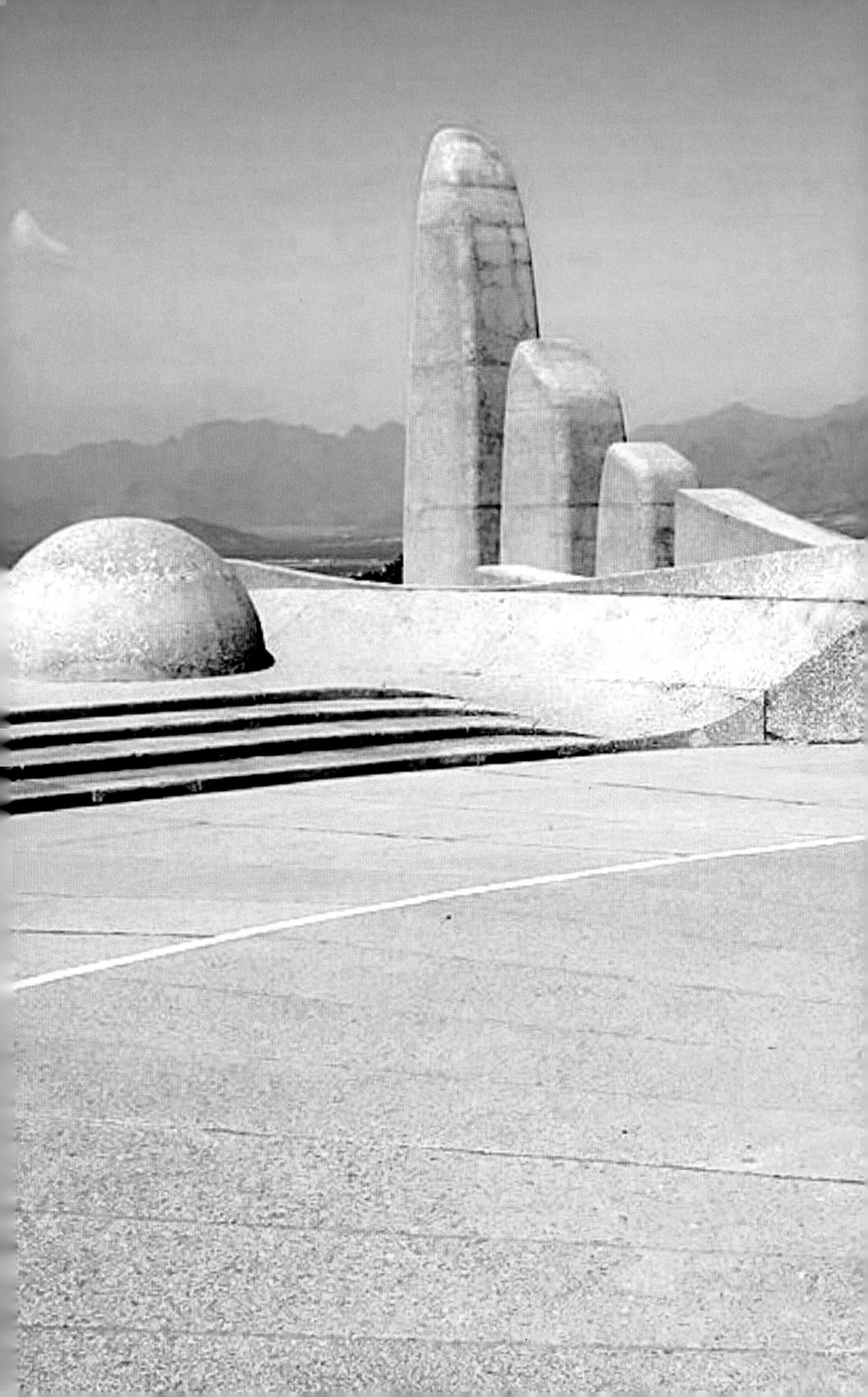

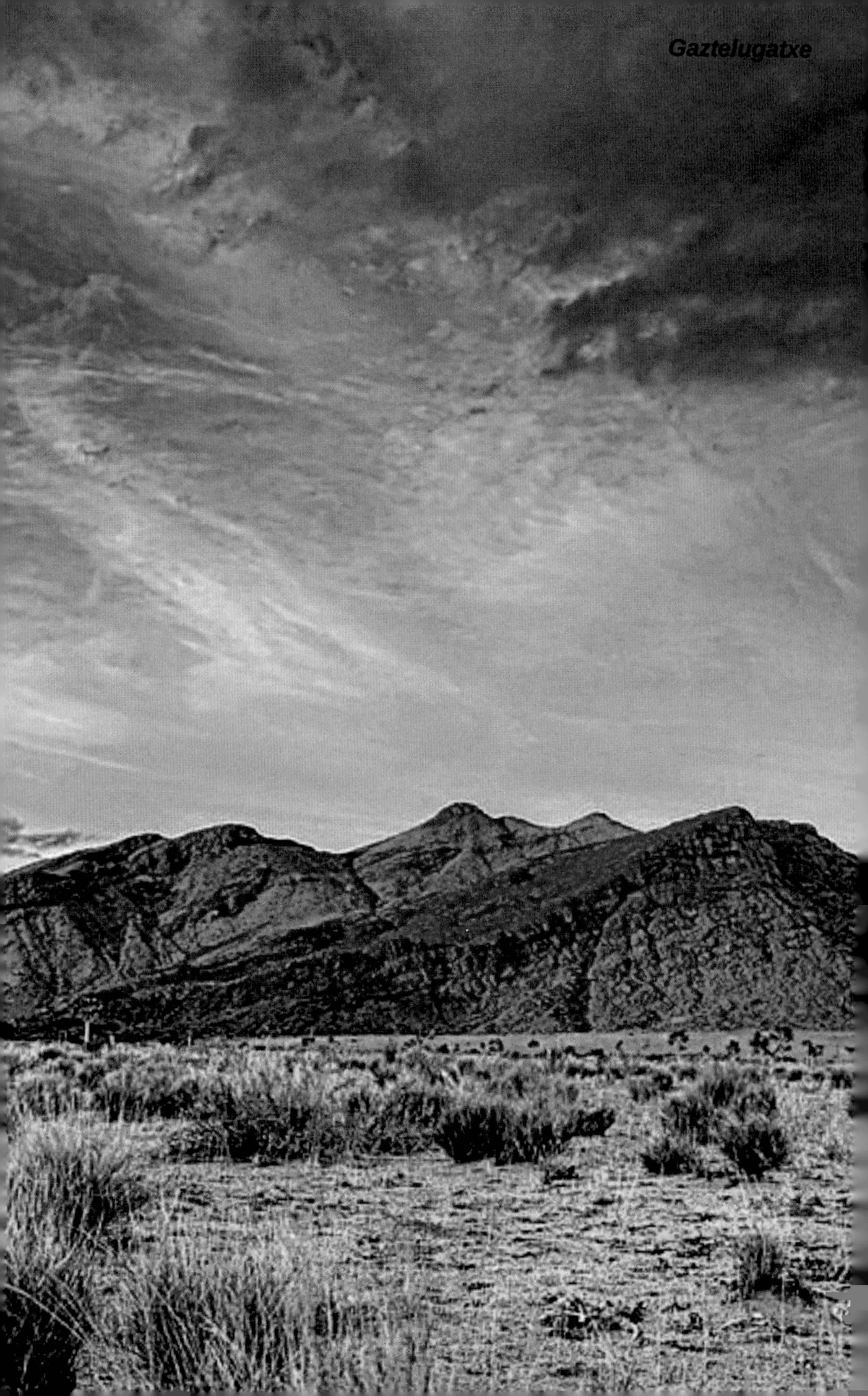
Gaztelugatxe

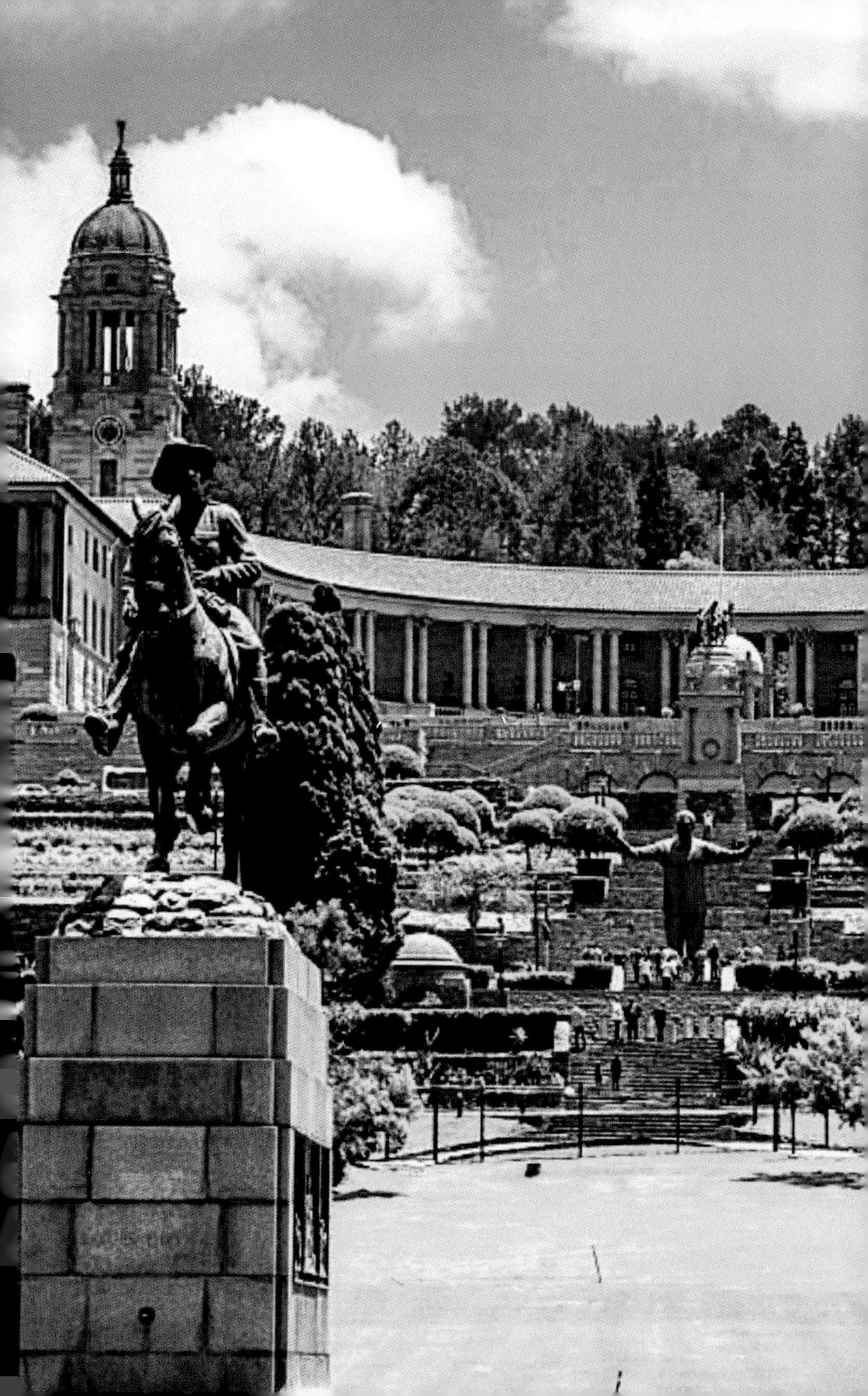

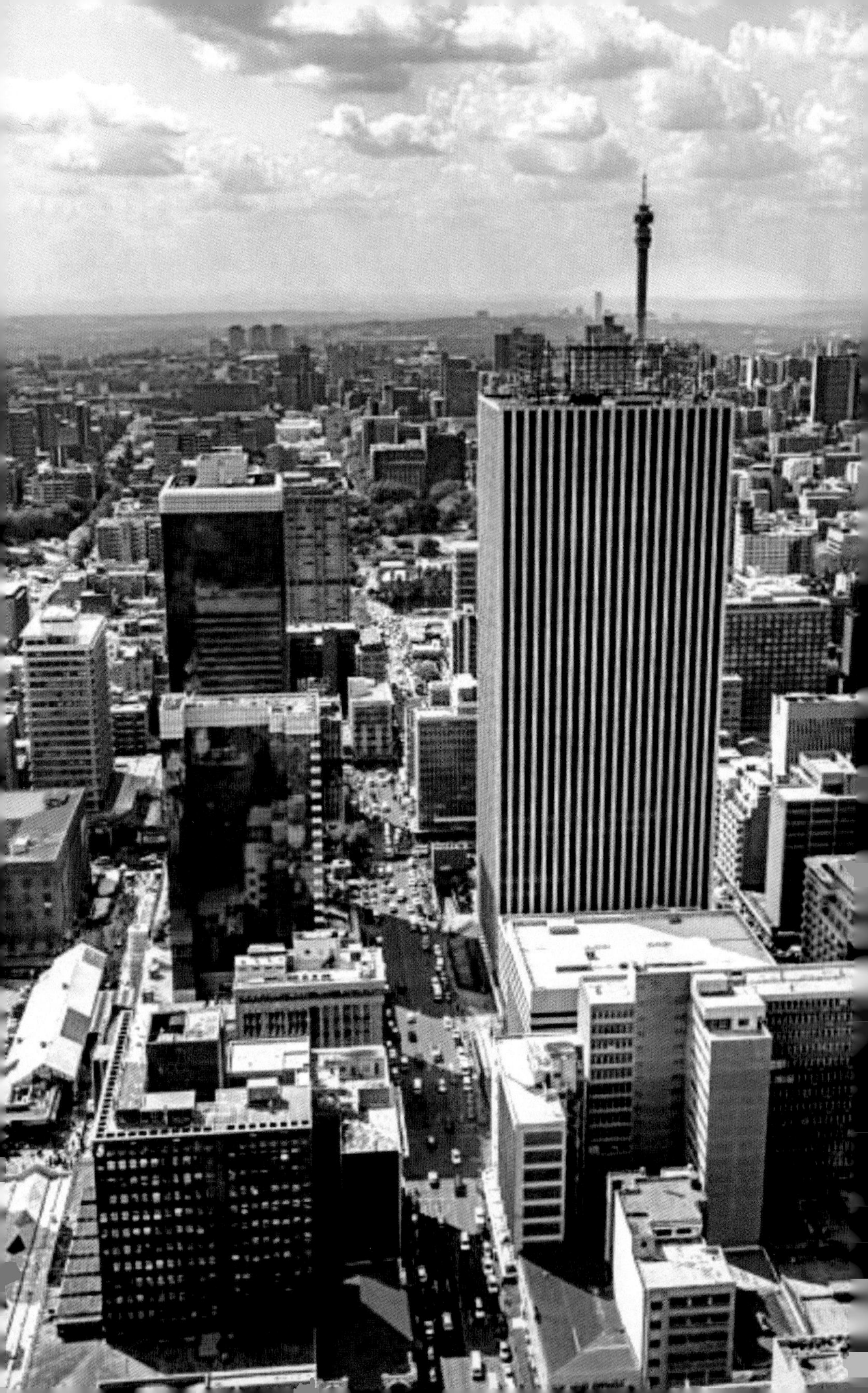

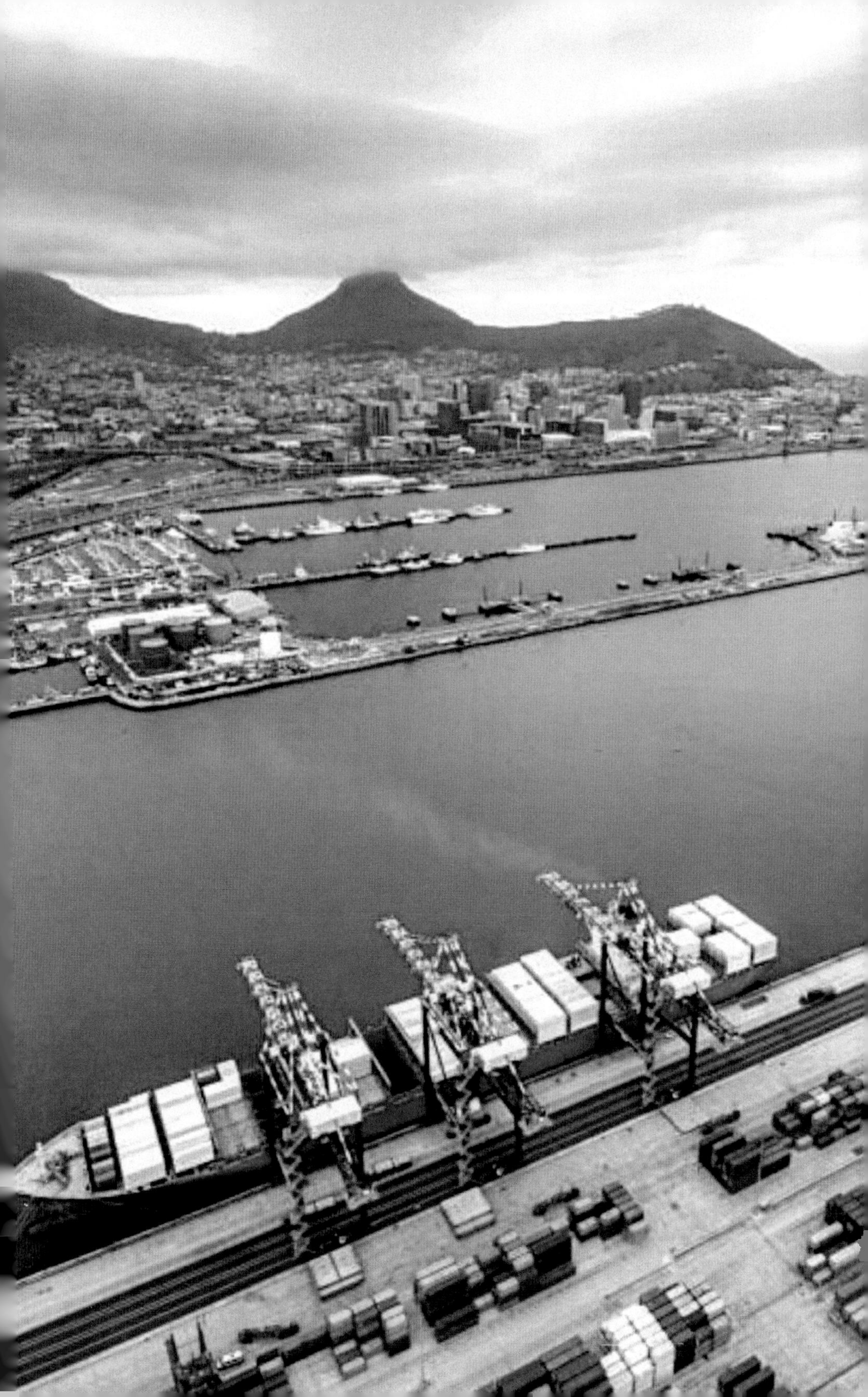

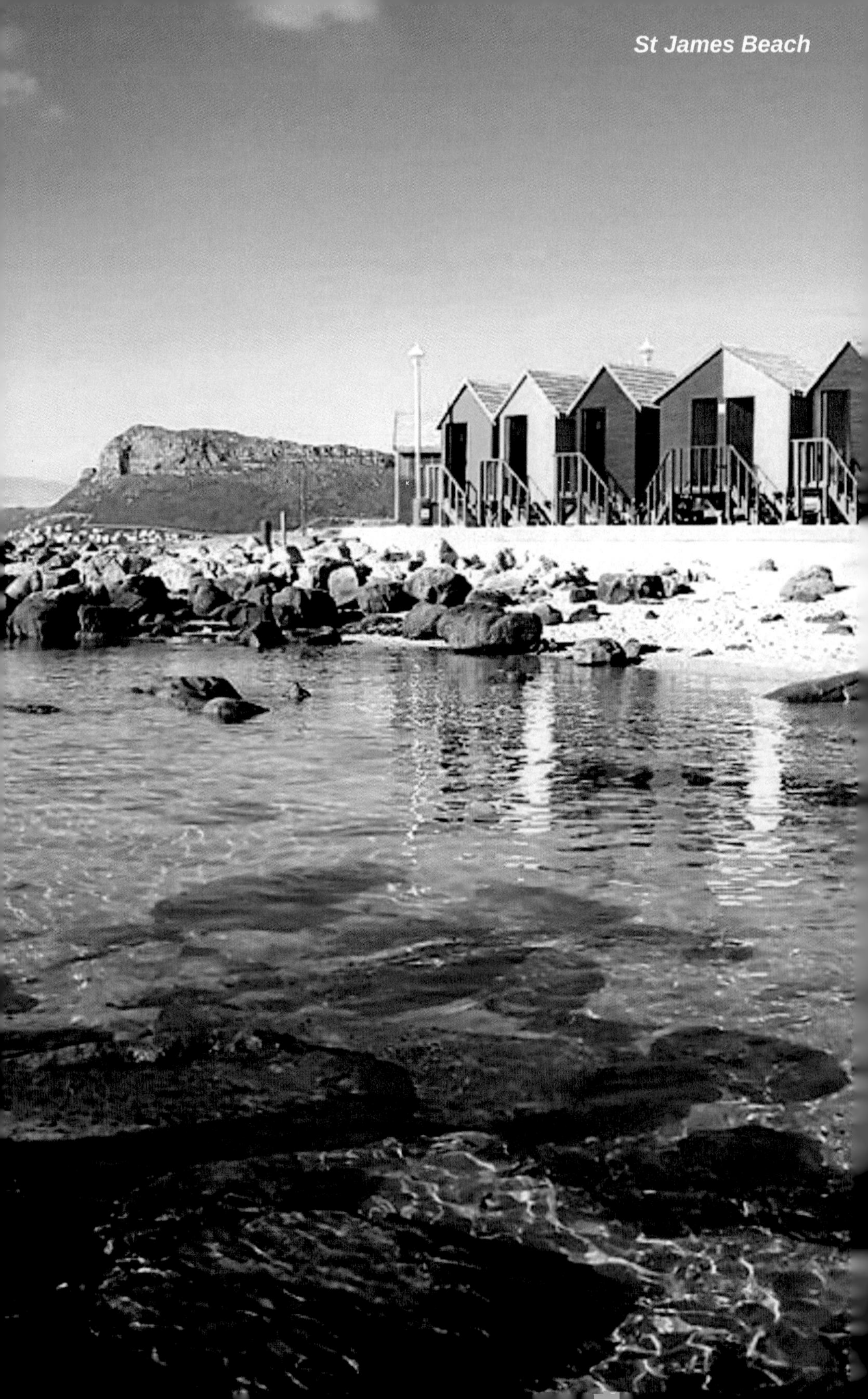
St James Beach

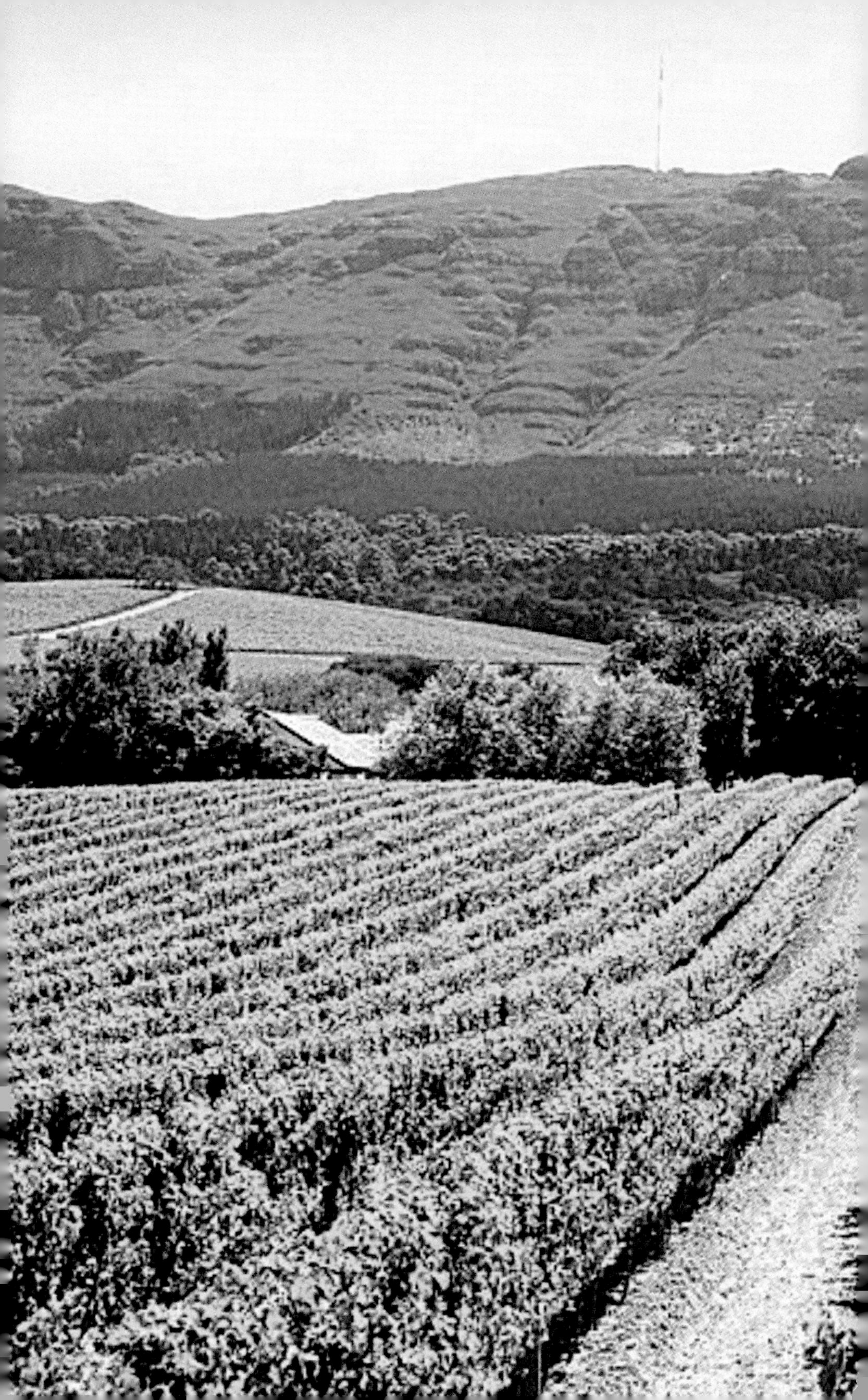

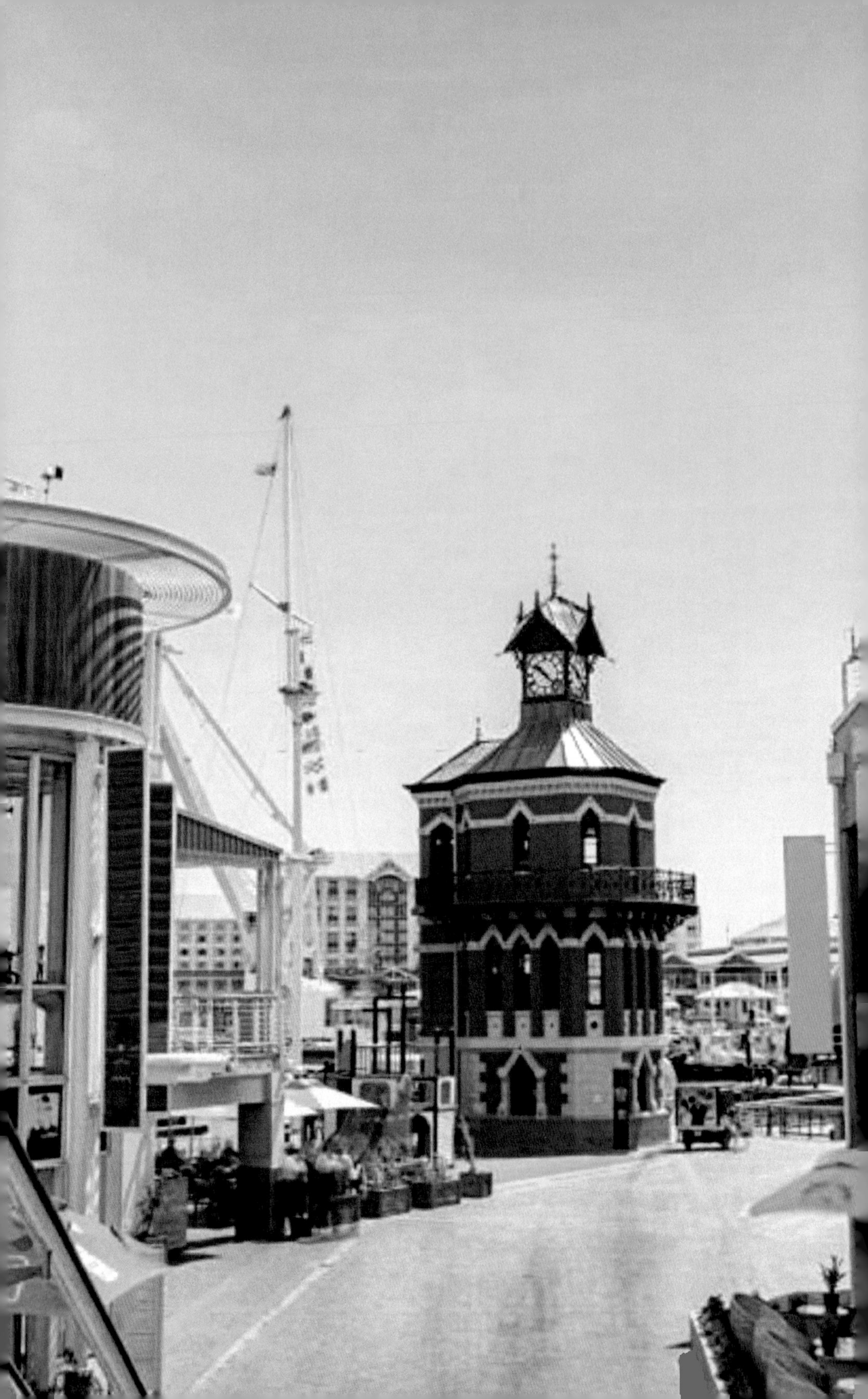

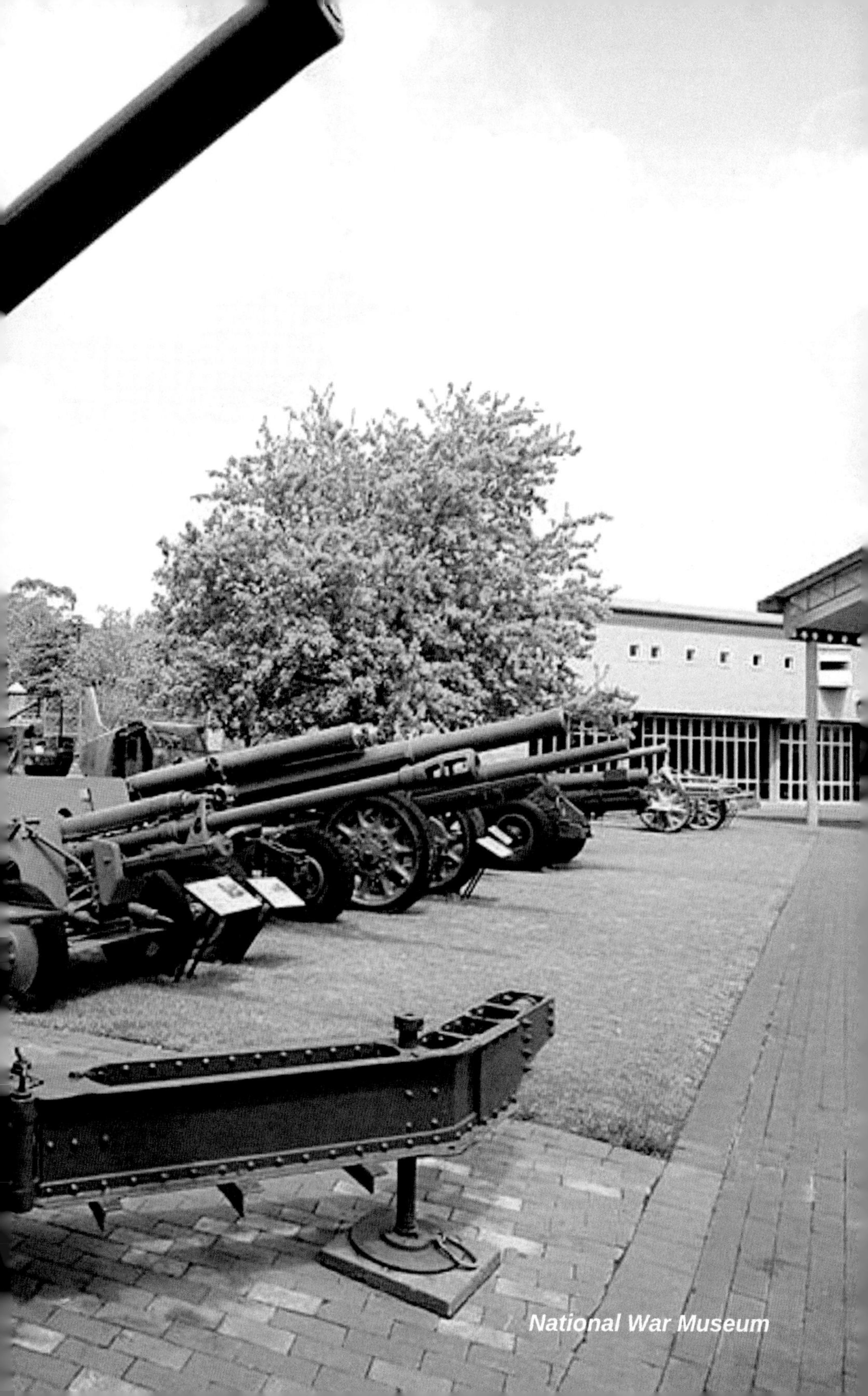

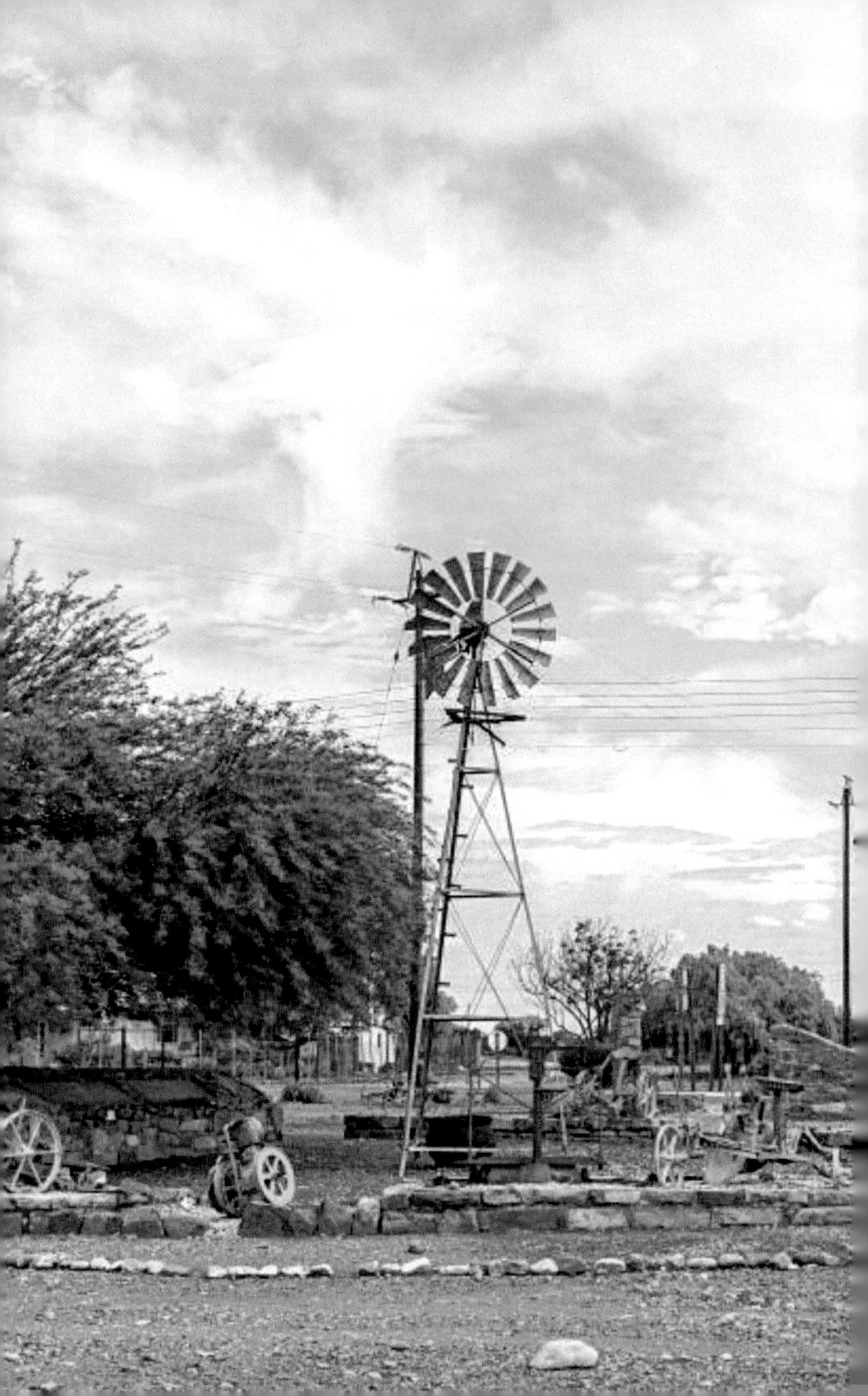

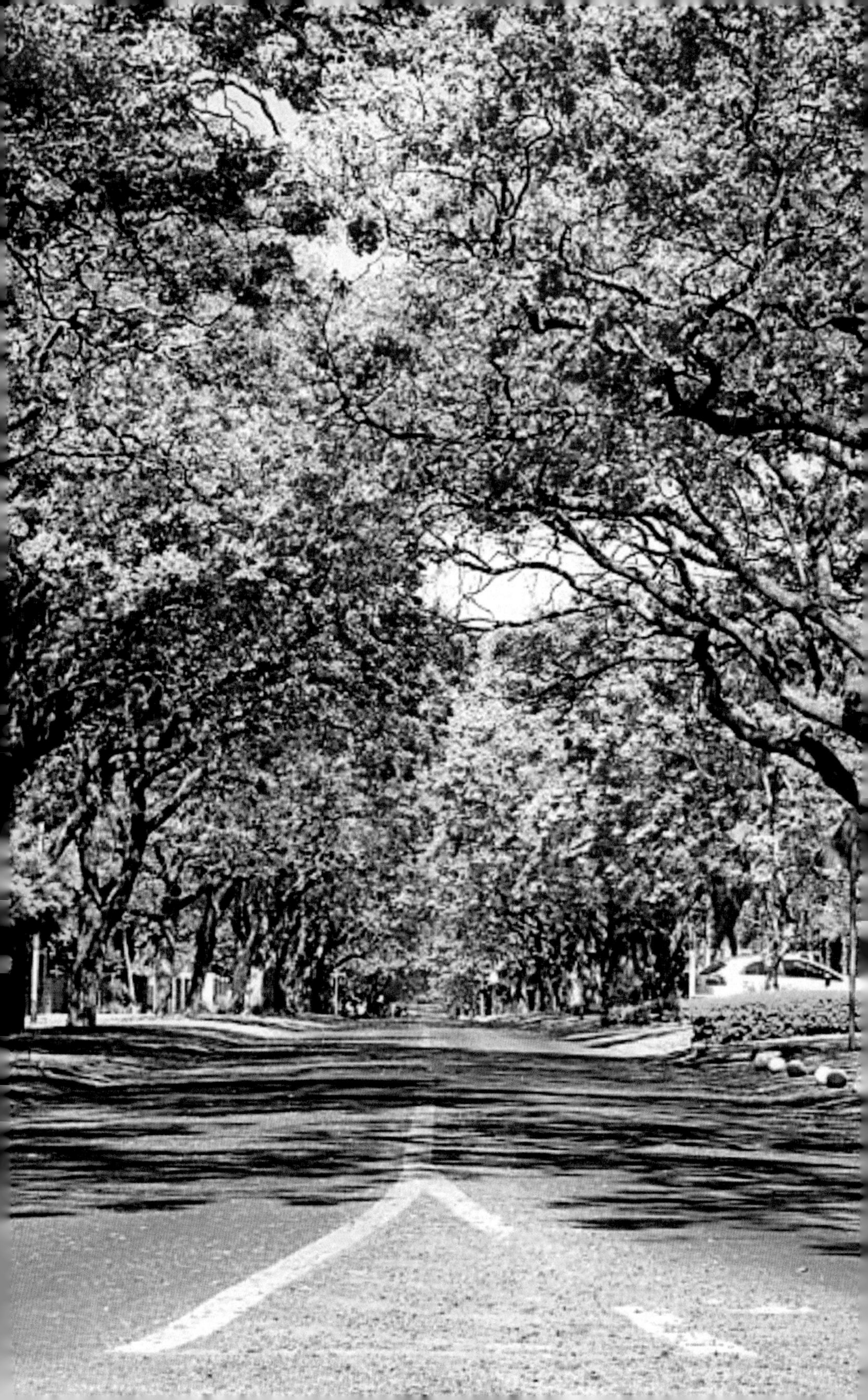

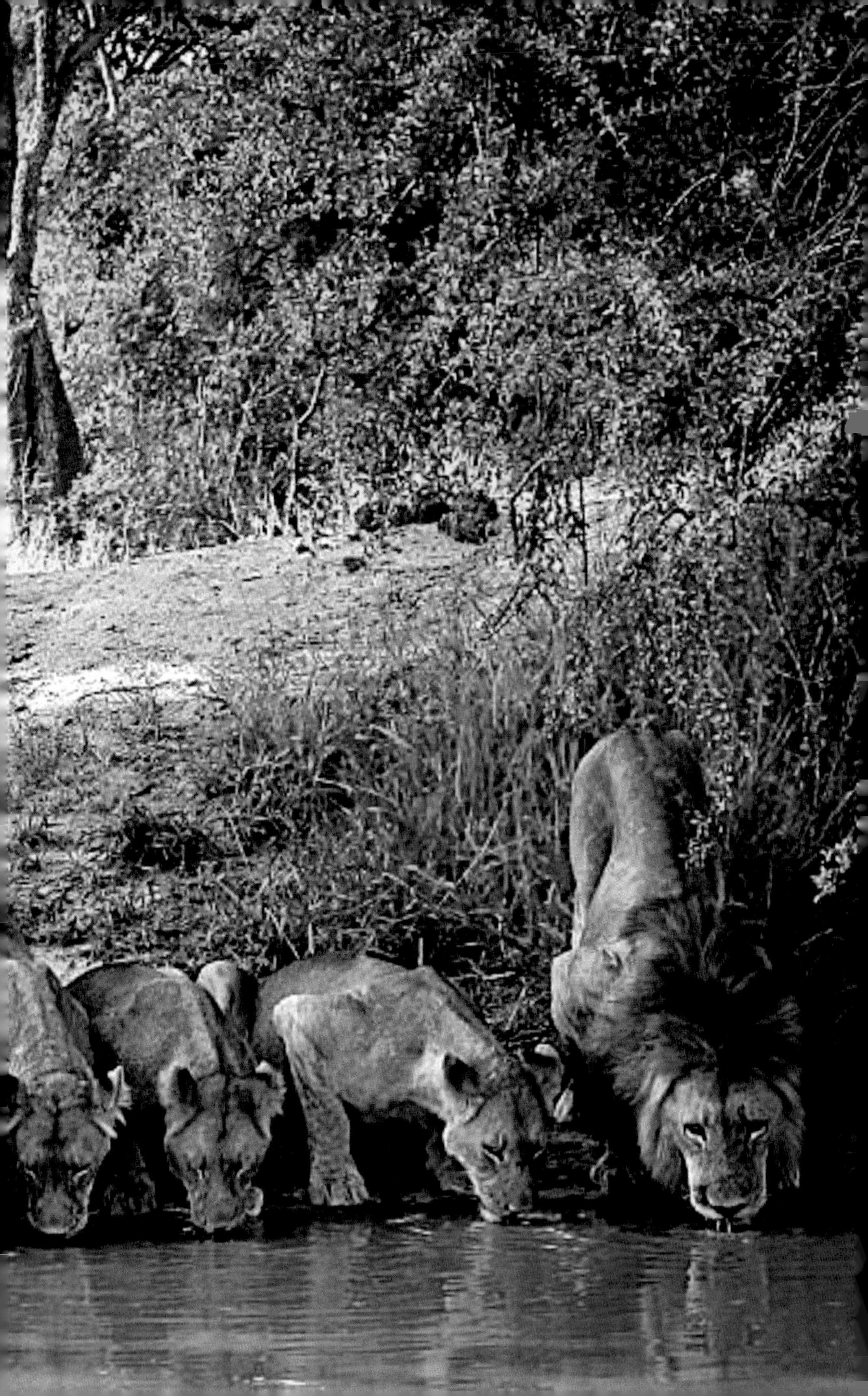

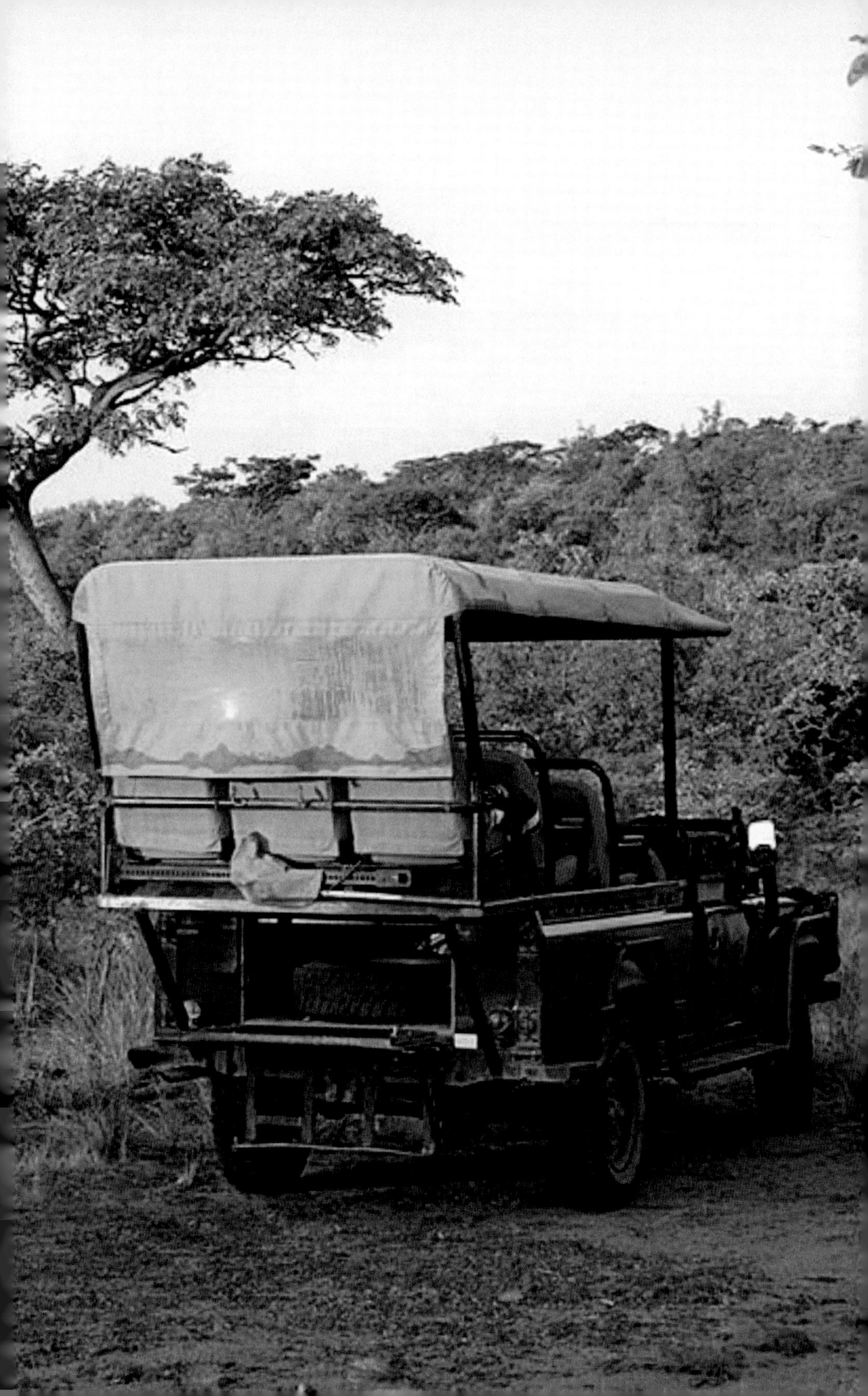

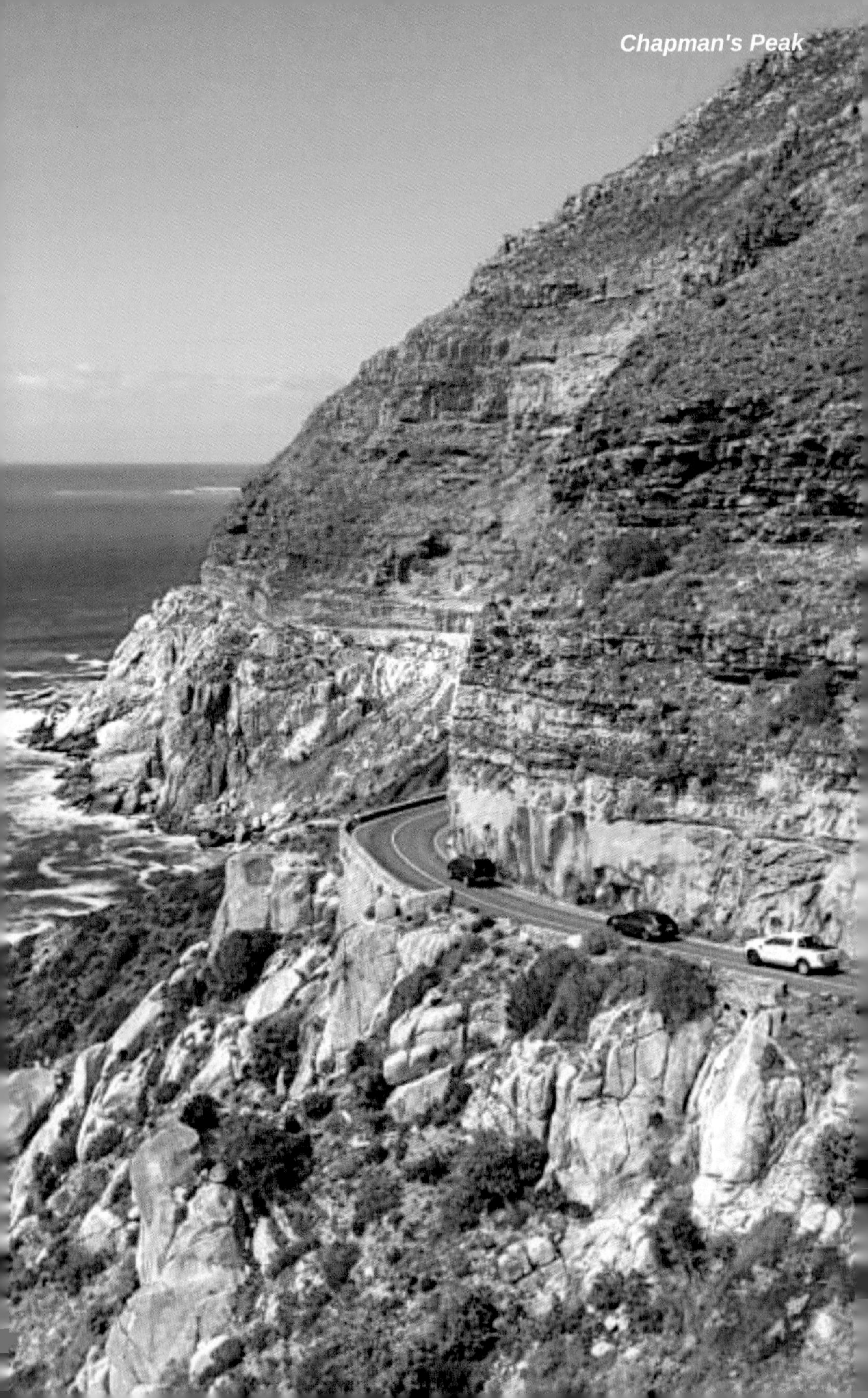
Chapman's Peak

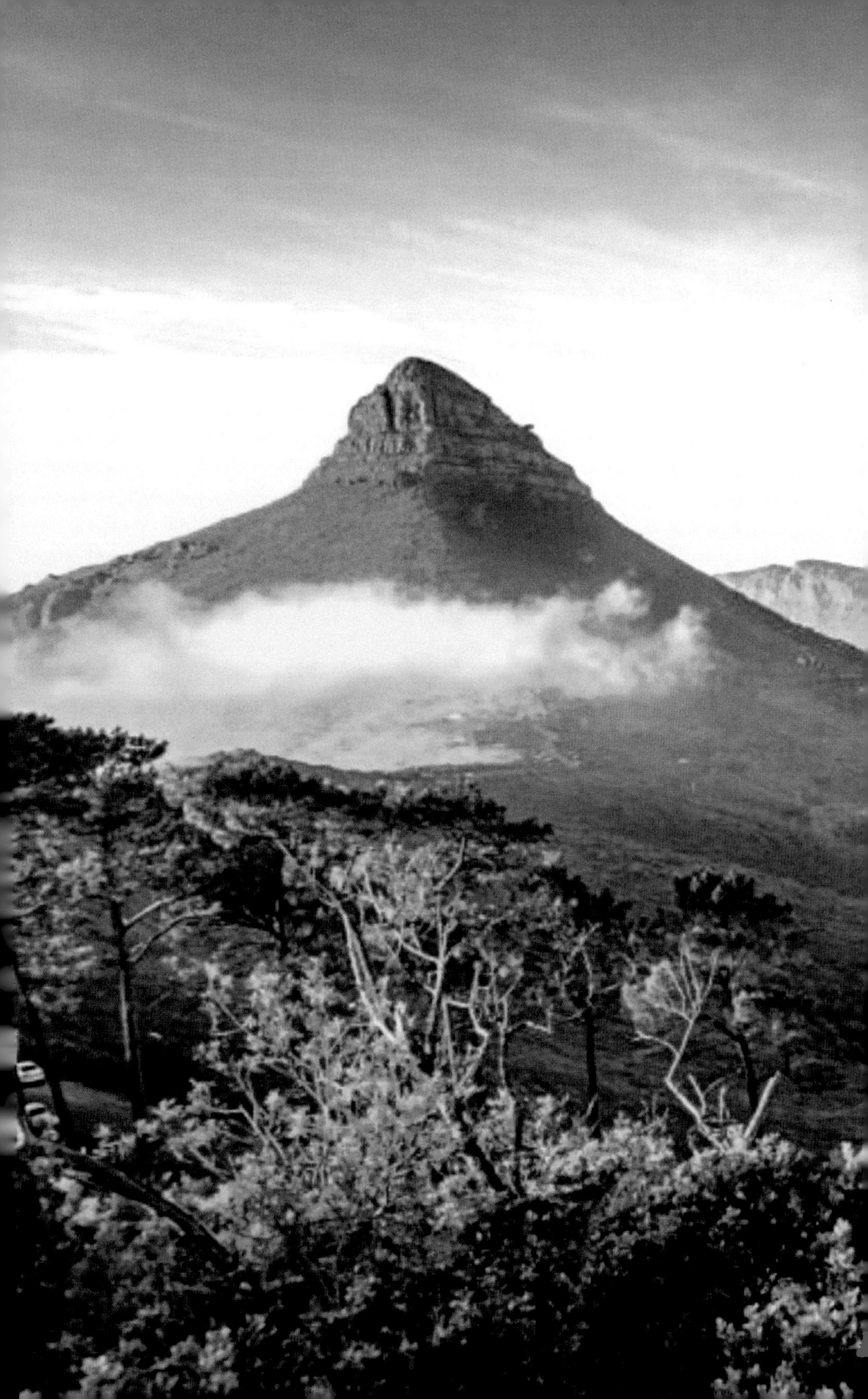

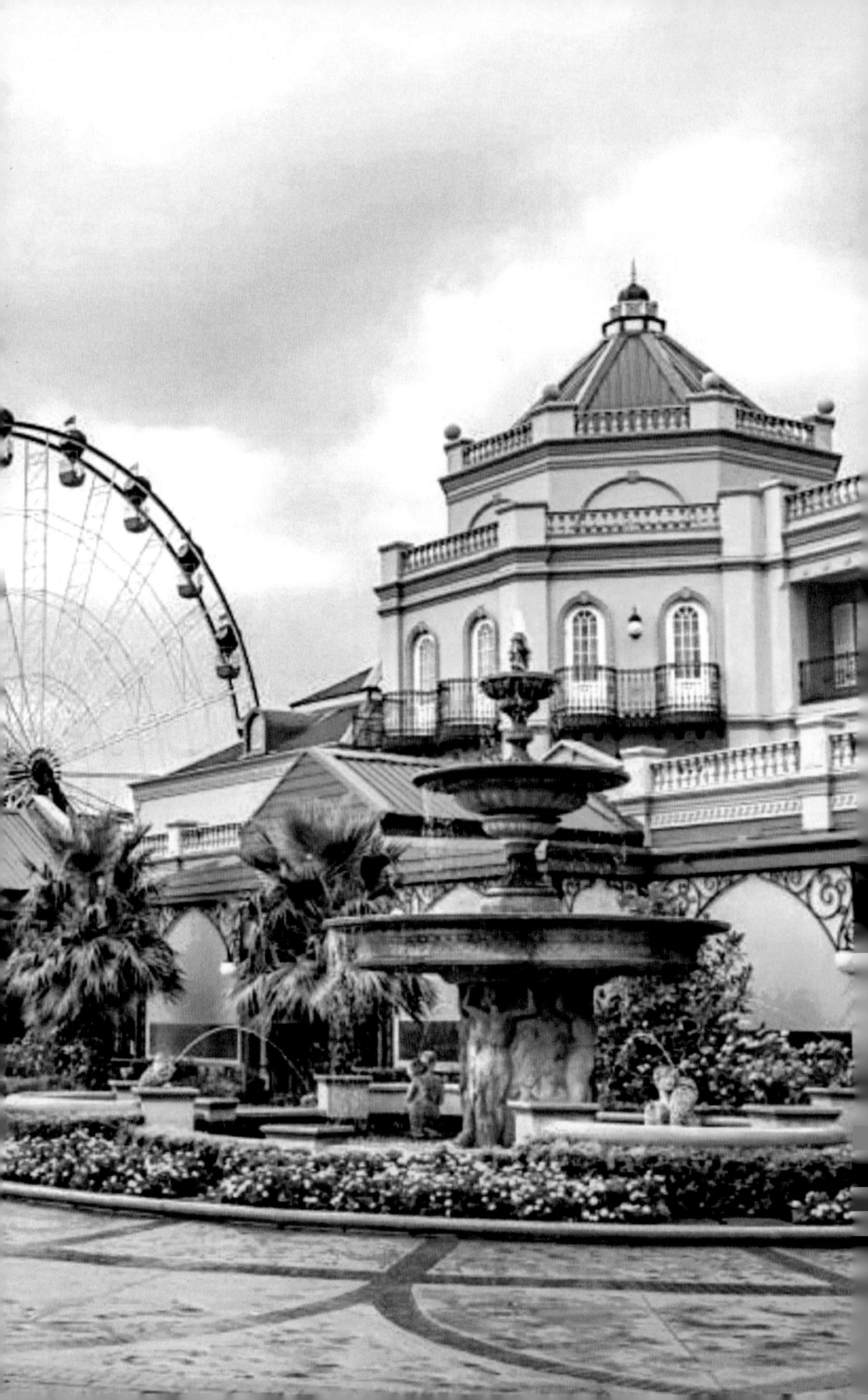

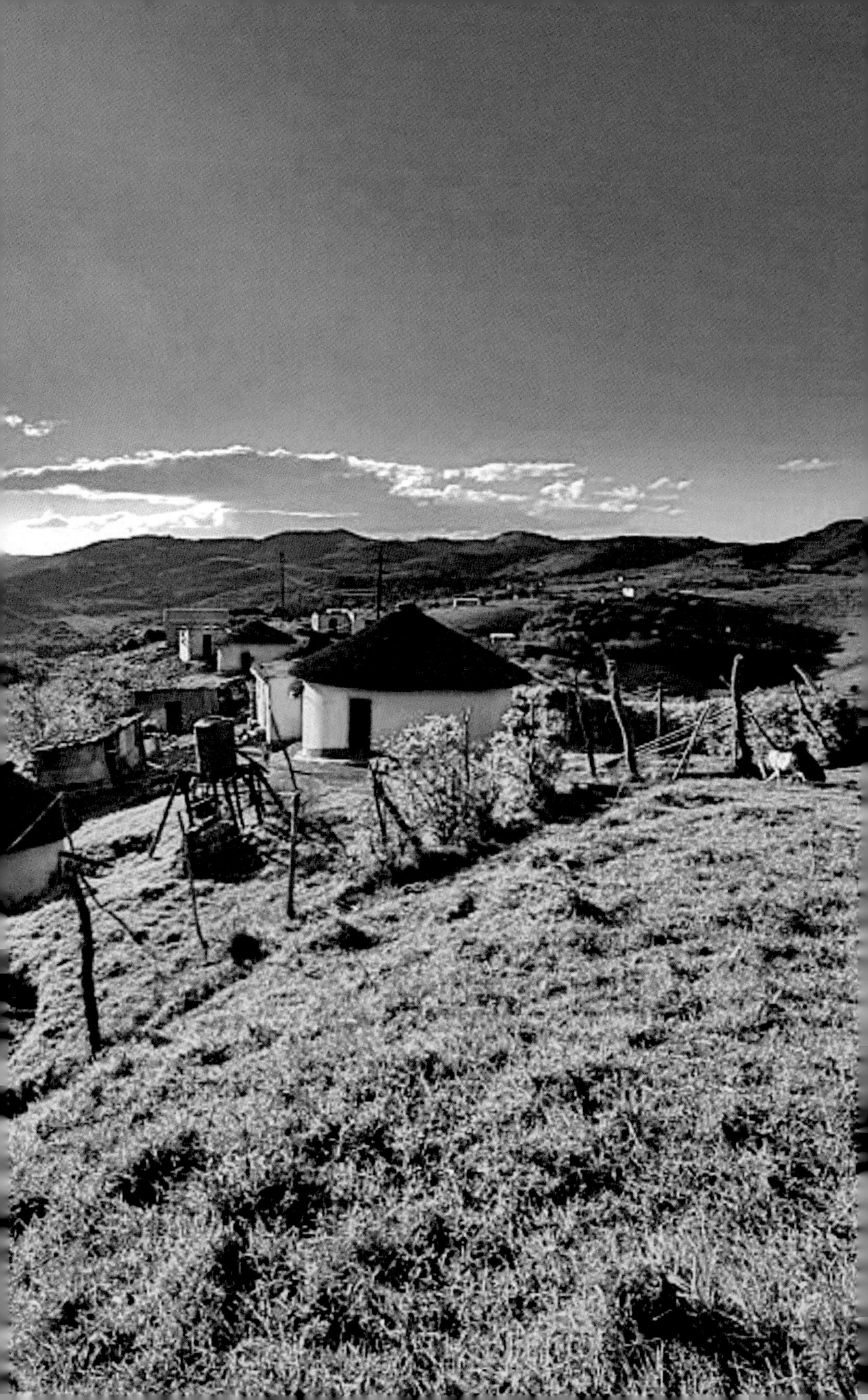

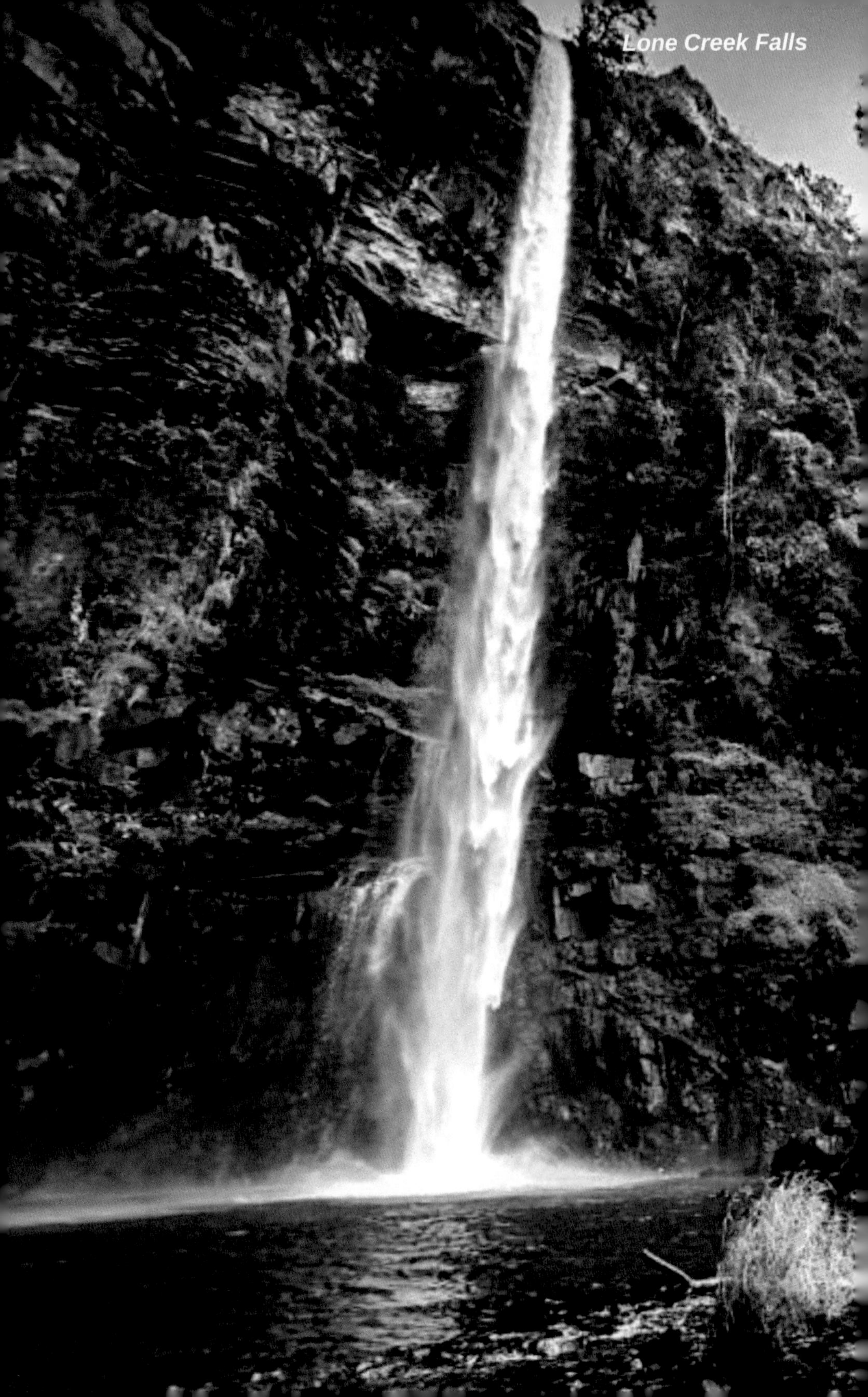
Lone Creek Falls

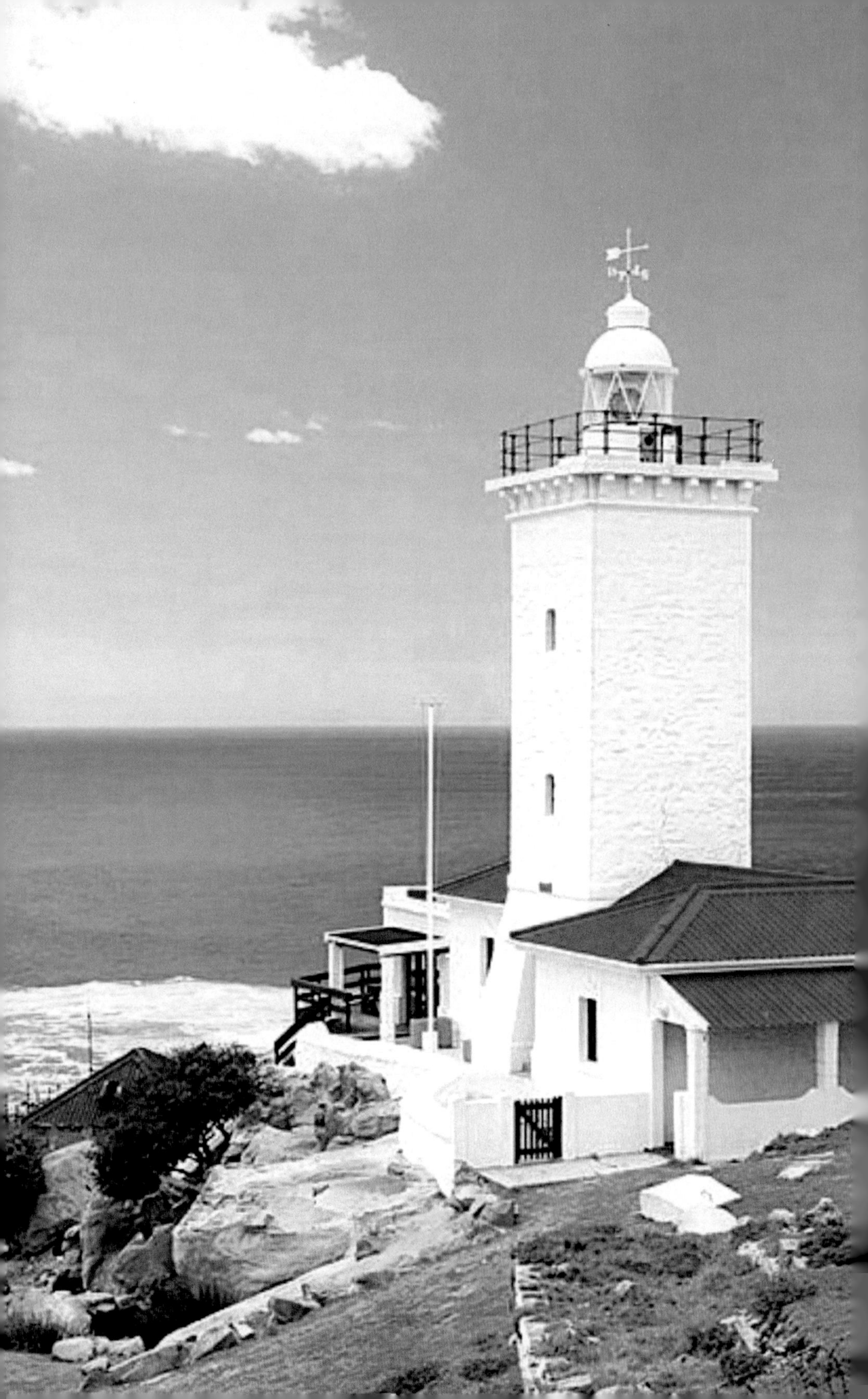

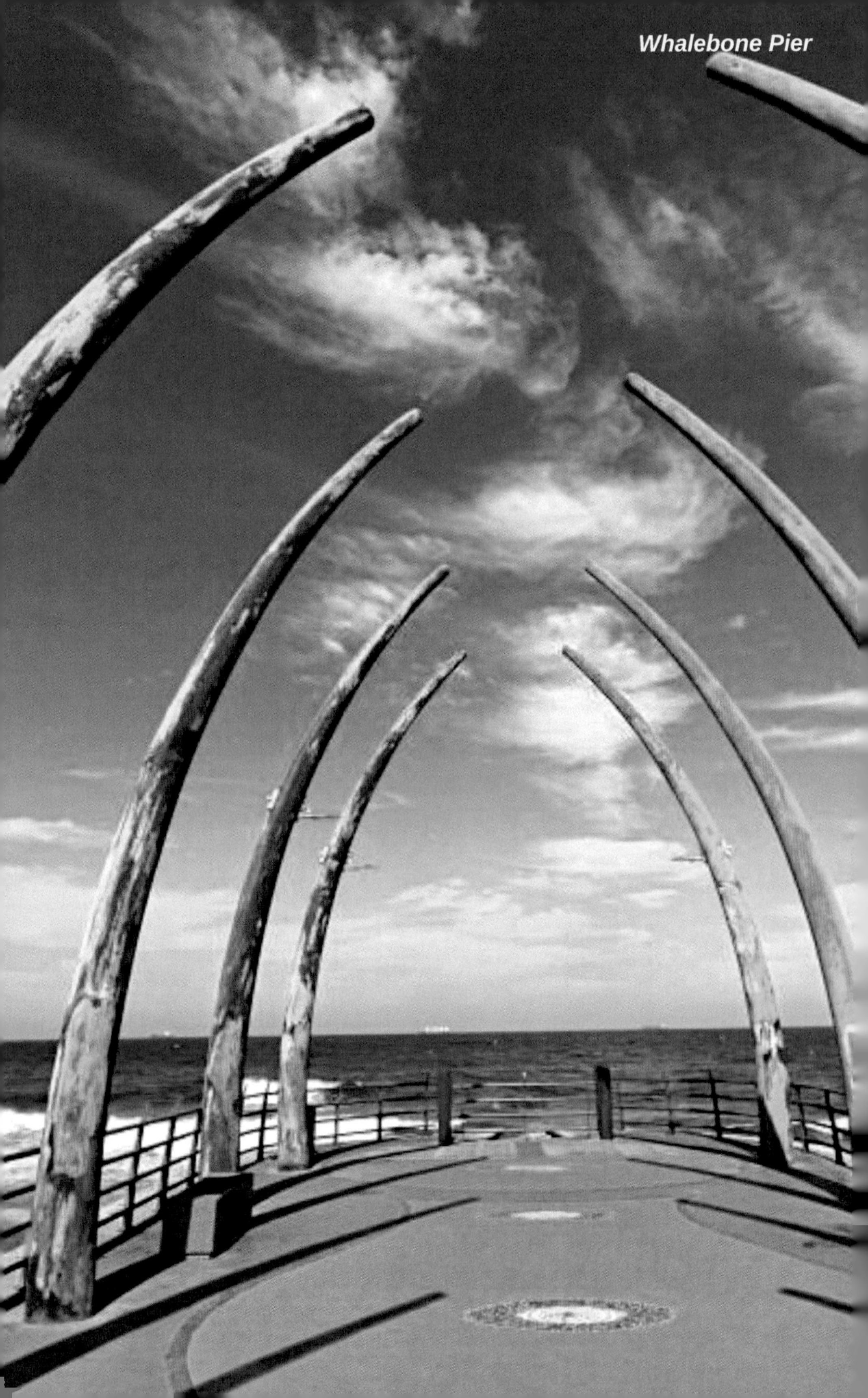

Whalebone Pier

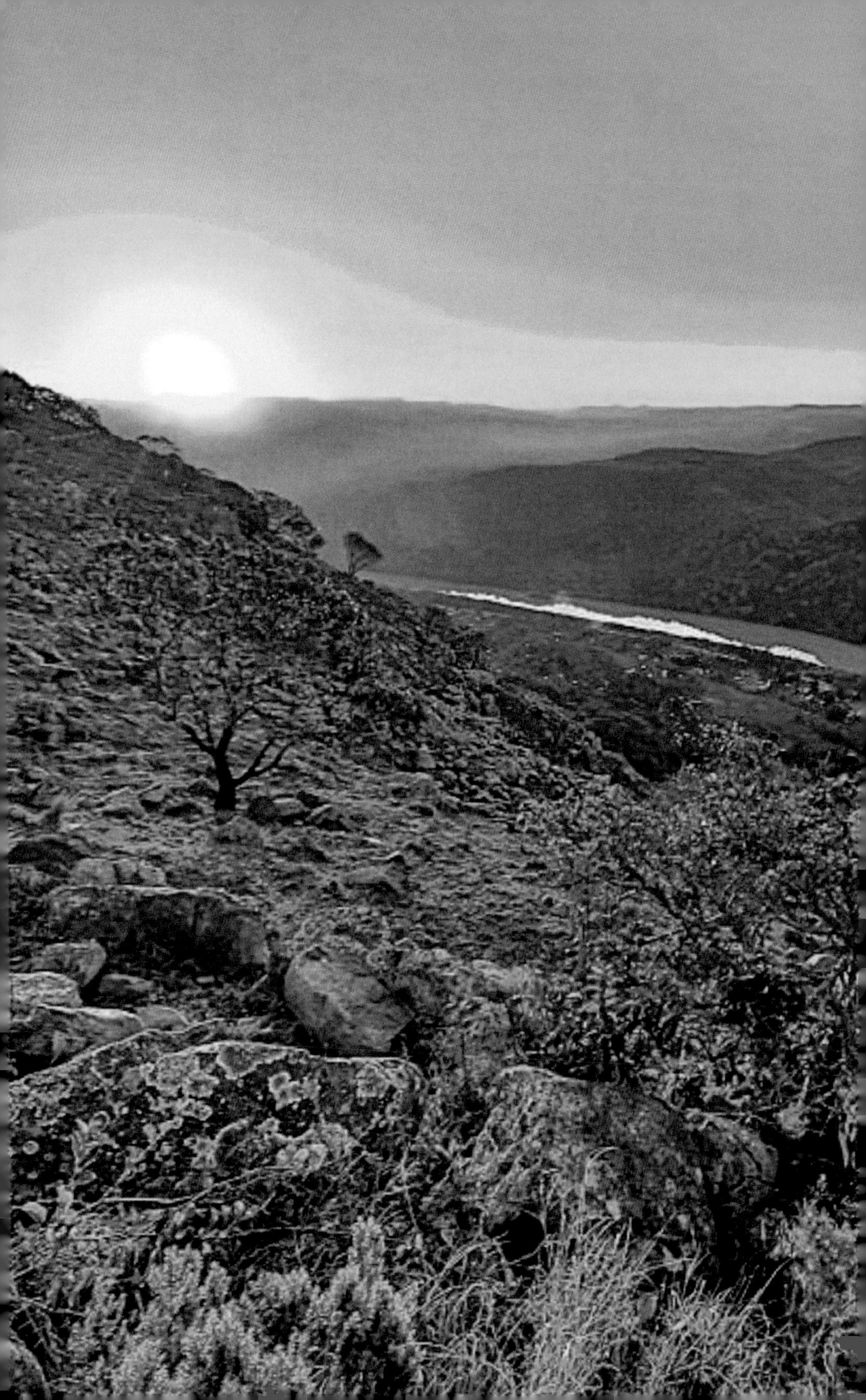

Made in the USA
Monee, IL
29 November 2022

18995752R00029